EXTRACORPOREAL LIFE SUPPORT

EXTRACORPOREAL LIFE SUPPORT

A Practical Guide
To
Extracorporeal Membrane Oxygenation
(ECMO)
and
Plasmapheresis

Jeffrey B. Sussmane M.D.

Copyright © 2012 by Jeffrey B. Sussmane M.D.

Library of Congress Control Number:		2009901549
ISBN:	Hardcover	978-1-4771-3318-7
	Softcover	978-1-4771-3317-0

All rights reserved. No part of this book may be reproduced or transmitted in any form or by any means, electronic or mechanical, including photocopying, recording, or by any information storage and retrieval system, without permission in writing from the copyright owner.

This book was printed in the United States of America.

To order additional copies of this book, contact:
Xlibris Corporation
1-888-795-4274
www.Xlibris.com
Orders@Xlibris.com
55968

Contents

Chapter 1 15
    Introduction 15
    Terminology and Techniques 16
    Venoarterial (VA) ECMO 17
        Considerations for VA Support 18
    Veno-Venous Bypass (VV) 18
        Considerations for VV Support 19
    Arteriovenous ECMO 19
        Artificial Placenta 20
    Indications and Criteria 21
    General Newborn Inclusion Criteria and Exclusion Criteria43,44 ... 22
        General Pediatric Inclusion and Exclusion Criteria 23
        Congenital Diaphragmatic Hernia43 24
        Selected Pediatric ECMO Diagnosis 25
        Cardiac and Septic Shock ECMO Inclusion Criteria 25
        Contraindications 26
    Special Considerations for the Pediatric ECMO Patient 26
        Adult Guidelines 27
        Outcomes 27
        Complications 28
    Physiology 29
    Physiology Formulas 30
        Oxygen Content 30
        Arteriovenous Oxygen Difference 30
        Factors that Affect Oxygen Content 31
        Factors That Affect Oxygen Delivery 38
    Oxygen Consumption 40
        Fick Principle 40
    Hemodynamics 44
Chapter 2 48
    Quality 48
        Technical Quality 48
        Process / Six Sigma 49

Performance Improvement	49
Functional Quality	50
SERVQUAL	51
Chapter 3	**53**
Precannulation	53
Precannulation Evaluation	54
Performance Improvement	55
Precannulation Process	55
Pre-ECMO Orders	56
Blood Bank Protocol	57
ECMO Specialist Responsibilities Prebypass	58
Additional Safety Checklist	60
Circuit Priming Process	60
Circuit Setup	61
Circuit Setup	61
Medtronic/Cobe Occulsion Pump	61
Crystalloid Priming and Setting Occlusion	64
Blood Prime	66
Device Safety Checklist:	70
Going on ECMO	72
Circuit Setup: Quadrox/Jostra HL—20 Centrifugal Pump	73
Crystalloid Priming	75
Blood Prime	77
Device Safety Checklist	81
Going on ECMO	83
Chapter 4	**85**
Medical Preparations Precannulation	85
ECMO Admission Orders	87
Chapter 5	**92**
Cannulation	92
Cannulation Process	92
Cannulation	92
Initiating VA Bypass	93
Initiating VV-ECMO Bypass	94
Primary Nurse Responsibility	94
Patient Management	95
Care of a Patient on ECMO	108
IV Fluids	110
ECMO Specialist Responsibilities	113
Taking Report	113
Restocking the ECMO Cart	115

  Blood Product Availability 115
  Blood Refrigerator 115
  Blood Bank Policy 115
  Fluid and Medication Administration 115
   A. Shopping List 123
   B. Procedure 123
Chapter 6. 126
  Hematologic Considerations on ECMO 126
 Newborn Considerations35, 36 126
  Vascular System 127
  Blood Flow / Stasis 127
  Coagulation Cofactors 127
  Clot Formation 128
  Passive Therapy 129
Chapter 7. 130
 Blood Product Administration 130
  Packed Red Blood Cells (PRBCs) 130
  Fresh Frozen Plasma (FFP) 131
  Platelets 131
  Calcium 133
  Magnesium 133
  Cryoprecipitate 134
  Albumin (5%) 134
  Albumin (25 %) 134
  Amicar 135
  Alteplase 136
  Recombinant Antithrombin III (rATIII) 136
  Heparin-Induced Thrombotic Thrombocytopenia 136
  Fibrin Glue 136
  Alternative Anticoagulation Therapies 137
 Coagulation Clinical Flow Sheet 140
 Anticoagulation Quality Management Tool 141
Chapter 8. 147
 Weaning and Idling for AV-ECMO for Infants 147
 Open-Bridge ECMO / Idling 148
 Weaning / Idling for VV-ECMO 150
 Trial Off / Decannulation 150
  Weaning / Trial-Off Note 152
  Decannulation 152
  Stinting 155

Chapter 9 158
Emergencies 158
Mechanical Circulatory Support 158
Perioperative Cardiac Surgery 158
Extracorporeal Membrane Oxygenation 160
Patient Emergencies 160
Sudden Cardiorespiratory Decompensation during ECMO 160
CPS and Cardiac Support for Emergencies 161
Emergency Decannulation 162
Acute Decompensation 163
Invasive Site Hemorrhage 166
Other Systems 166
Air Emboli 167
Patent Ductus Arteriosus 168

Chapter 10 170
Mechanical Emergencies on ECMO 170
Circuit Emergencies 170
Taking a Patient Off Pump for an Emergency 170
Changing the Oxygenator (Medtronic) 170
Priming New Oxygenator (Medtronic) 171
Blood Priming New Oxygenator 171
Placing New Oxygenator in Line 172
Priming New Heat Exchanger 172
Setup 172
Blood Prime 173
Replace Heat Exchanger 173

Chapter 11 174
Plasmapheresis 174
Introduction 174
Common Indications 175
Principles of TPE Operation 175
Specific Considerations for the ECMO Circuit 177
Specific Humoral 178

Chapter 12 180
Physiology of Plasmapheresis 180
Physiologic Considerations 180
Circuit Priming 183
Calculation of Fluid Balance 183
Anticoagulation 184
Complications 185

Chapter 13 187
    Nursing and Plasmapheresis 187
    Patient Nursing Care of ECMO TPE Patient 187
Chapter 14 189
    Apheresis Specialist Training and Competencies 189
    Planned Maintenance 190
    Apheresis Checklist 190
    Apheresis Specialist 190
Chapter 15 193
    ECMO Certification 193
    ECMO Specialist Competencies 193
        Module I—Didactic 193
        Module II—Water Labs 193
        Module III—Animal Labs 193
        Module IV—Clinical Orientation 194
    ECMO Specialist Commitment 194
        Recertification—Annual 194
        ECMO Specialist Training Program 194
        Module I—Didactic 194
        Module II—Water Labs 195
        Module III—Clinical Orientation 196
Chapter 16 198
    Final Clinical Water Lab 1 198
    Final Clinical Water Lab II 206
Abbreviation List 209
Bibliography 211
Index 217

Acknowledgments

Extracorporeal life support has and will take health care into new and magnificent opportunities. May this practical guide provide assistance to anyone embarking on this noble cause, and may these words provide some evidence to the many extraordinarily gifted individuals who began to see this light and have followed it. The ability to provide life-saving care to a child and their family is one of the greatest blessings that may be bestowed. My sincere gratitude to the countless amazingly dedicated colleagues who have allowed me to learn with them.

Thank you.

Disclaimer

The author and publisher remind the reader that this is only a compilation of clinical experience as it relates to a highly complex and unique field in medicine. Presentations and patients may appear similar, but individual responses are unpredictable. This is just a guide that must be utilized within a highly organized environment with constant supervision by experienced individuals. The advice given is hopefully helpful but does not suggest results.

CHAPTER 1

Introduction

Huang Di, the Yellow Emperor of China in the middle of the third millennium BCE, wrote one of the earliest and most complete texts of medicine. The *Neijing* or *Yellow Emperor's Classic of Medicine* is an extraordinary collection of wisdom seeking to balance and improve one's natural life force.[1] The western world thanks Anaximenes of Miletus who first described air in the sixth century BCE.[2] Greece continued to dominate the advancement of medicine, and in the fifth century BCE, they created a clear separation away from divine medicine, and observation theory was established. The Greeks are credited with establishing therapies to balance, remove, and replace circulating substances in the body.[3] There may have been several physicians referred to as Hippocrates, but he is credited with the first reference to the four "humours:" blood, phlegm, black bile, and yellow bile.[3] Ctesibius of Alexandria provided the first scientific description of pneumatics in the third century BCE.[4] *Pneumatica* (πνευματικά) was first described as the study of devices operated by air or water pressure.[4] The Buddha (c. 250 BCE) is credited with the Aryuvedic concept of disease caused by an imbalance of air, bile, and phlegm.[5] The foundation of modern medicine is found in this commonality of ancient thought. This is all the more striking when we review the advanced applications of current extracorporeal technology. A more modern reference to pneumatic chemistry "is a term most-closely identified with an area of scientific research of the seventeenth, eighteenth, and early nineteenth centuries. Important goals of this work were an understanding of the physical properties of gases and how they relate to chemical reactions."[6]

Richard Lower published his seminal work *Tractatus de Corde* in 1669 where he describes "the observation that blackish blood, which reached the lungs through the pulmonary artery, returned to the heart by the pulmonary veins a beautiful red color."[7] John Jacob Abel, known as the father of pharmacology, is credited with the development of a vividiffusion apparatus, the first artificial kidney. He was assisted by Rowntree and Turner and first demonstrated this device at the physiological congress in Groningen in 1914.[8, 9] Willem Johan Kolff, also from Groningen and known as the father of the artificial organ, is credited with observing the oxygenation of blood as it passed over the celloidin membrane of the secret dialysis machine he was developing in 1944.[10, 11] Kolff described one of the earliest uses of this membrane in 1956 and is known for the assistance he gave to his fellow, Robert Jarvick, in the design and implantation of the first artificial human heart.[12, 13] This decade saw many technological advances in cardiopulmonary support. John Gibbon is credited with the first application of cardiopulmonary support in 1954.[14] The refinement of the membrane oxygenator by Clowes in 1956, enabled prolonged cardiopulmonary bypass to become feasible.[15] A more thorough review of modern cardiopulmonary support may be enjoyed with the work of Lillehei.[16] Adams and Skoog are credited with the first clinical application of plasmapheresis in 1957.[17]

The modern concept of an intensive care unit began when Hill et al. successfully applied a cardiopulmonary device to a patient for three days in 1972.[18] This early extracorporeal success disseminated quickly throughout the modern intensive care unit and, unfortunately, was overenthusiastically applied. Poorly designed studies and lack of comprehensive training doomed the initial application of extracorporeal life support.[19] The failure of an NIH study might have completely stopped the clinical application of ECMO were it not for Bartlett et al. who successfully applied ECMO to the term *newborn population*.[20,21] The advancement of ECMO as an accepted worldwide technology became solidified with the formation of a voluntary academic consortium, ELSO, in 1989. This has galvanized the clinical practice of ECMO. ELSO is responsible for creating and maintaining one of the largest international clinical databases in the world with over 46,000 patients and 145 active centers. Focused on a mission to improve patient care through collaboration, the database now boosts almost 25,000 newborn cases with an 85% ECMO survival rate with a 75% rate of discharge for newborns previously moribund.[22]

Terminology and Techniques

ECMO stands for extracorporeal membrane oxygenation. The first are Latin-derived terms: *extra* meaning outside and *corporeal* meaning body. A membrane oxygenator is a device that has an artificial surface that allows oxygen and carbon dioxide gas to diffuse across the surface. A gradient is created across this artificial membrane between a gas mixture of oxygen and carbon dioxide and the blood. This allows the membrane to exchange oxygen and carbon dioxide with the blood and act as an artificial lung to deliver oxygen to and remove carbon dioxide from the blood. This artificial lung significantly reduces or may eliminate the need for the use of a machine called a ventilator. A ventilator is a machine that is used to provide artificial breathing to support patients during life-threatening respiratory failure. ECMO is performed by extracting blood from the central circulation and returning the blood to the central circulation with a plastic tubing circuit. There is a pump placed in the circuit. This pump circulates the blood through the circuit, from the patient's body through the artificial lung, through a rewarming device, and back to the patient. This pump can also perform as an artificial heart if necessary. ECMO technology allows the lung and, if necessary, the heart to rest and heal. ECMO may also avoid the iatrogenic injury that may be associated with the use of artificial ventilation and chemical support of the heart in critical situations.

ECLS stands for extracorporeal life support. This refers to variations in the application of an artificial device outside of the body. This term primarily applies to artificial cardiorespiratory support but may include other technologies such as plasmapheresis and artificial hepatic support. This term does not frequently refer to dialysis for renal failure. Further clarification is below.

Although this is an exciting therapy, it should only be offered to the appropriate patient population in the appropriate institution. Because of the intensive nature and expertise required to safely offer this therapy, it must be offered in regionalized ECMO centers with extensive experience, research, and follow-up programs. Early consultation with regionalization and transportation has dramatically improved and maintained an exceptional level of care and survival for the sickest of ICU patients.

Venoarterial (VA) ECMO

Venoarterial ECMO is the term used to describe ECLS by the drainage of blood from the central venous system, pumped through an artificial lung, and returned to the body into the arterial system. The blood may be acquired from a single or multiple large central veins or a cardiac chamber directly. The internal jugular vein is typically used for the venous access. The internal carotid artery is typically used for the arterial return. The blood returned to the arterial system is pressurized to systemic pressures and rewarmed. It is fully oxygenated and has the carbon dioxide removed to normal arterial values.

The advantages of this mode of ECLS are that it may provide full support for the cardiac and pulmonary systems. During VA bypass, the pulmonary artery pressure drops and decreases the intrapulmonary artery capillary pressure. This lowers the intracapillary hydrostatic water loss, which also lowers the intrapulmonary water volume. The ligation of the internal carotid artery is seen as a long-term disadvantage, although there are no reported sequlae.[23,24] There is the potential disadvantage of the showering of emboli directly into the arterial system. Systemic hyperoxia may also occur during VA bypass. VA bypass is designed to provide supersystemic cardiac output and thus oxygen delivery for conditions that require a greater degree of support. This clinical condition is often recognized when the ratio of oxygen delivery (DO_2) to oxygen consumption (VO_2), DO_2/VO_2, drops below 3/1 (unpublished data). To date, over sixteen thousand VA cases have been reported to the ELSO international registry with a 72% survival.[22]

Considerations for VA Support

Advantages of VA ECMO include support of heart and lung failure and thus enable complete cardiopulmonary support. Since VA ECMO may provide complete cardiopulmonary support, significant native cardiac function is not essential. This allows cardiac and pulmonary rest. While on VA bypass, the pulmonary artery pressures drops and the pulmonary capillary filtration pressure decreases, which diminishes the extravascular pulmonary water, thus favoring improvement of the oncotic gradient and extravascular pulmonary volume.

Disadvantages of VA ECMO include arterial and venous ligation of blood vessels from the brain. Air bubbles, particles, or embolism may be introduced into the circuit and can be infused directly into the arterial circulation. There is also an increased potential for hyperoxia.

Veno-Venous Bypass (VV)

Kolobow first described successful long-term (one week) VV bypass in 1969.[25] This form of VV bypass utilized two separate venous catheters. Central venous blood is directed through a pump, and an oxygenator was rewarmed and returned to another central vein. This has the advantage of sparing the carotid artery and reducing the threat of direct arterial emboli. There may be a technical challenge in isolating two vessels and obtaining adequate flow from two vessels. Zwischenberger first described the successful use of a single double-lumen catheter in 1985.[26] A single double-lumen catheter placed in the internal jugular vein eliminates the need for two vessel cannulation and has been designed to provide adequate flow for many clinical circumstances. VV bypass provides a significant improvement in the oxygenation of the pulmonary arterial blood. The improved oxygenation of the mixed venous circulation improves pulmonary and cardiac function while reducing iatrogenic injury during ventilation. This also subsequently improves systemic oxygenation. It is well suited for primary respiratory failure but improves systemic function with the reduction or elimination of hypoxia. This form of bypass may again require conversion to VA bypass if the DO2/VO2 ratio remains below 3:1. (See further explanation in ECMO physiology section.) To date, over five thousand VV double-lumen cases have been reported to ELSO with an 85% survival.[22]

Considerations for VV Support

Newborn VV ECMO may be accomplished with a single 14 Fr., a double-lumen catheter. Catheters are available that are rated up to 600 cc/min flow. This flow will support the oxygen delivery of an infant up to 4.5 kg as long as the oxygen delivery / oxygen consumption ratio remains above 2/1 (see further explanation in ECMO physiology section).

1. VV ECMO does not require carotid artery ligation.
2. Cephalic drainage may be required.
3. Carbon dioxide elimination of 3-6 cc/kg/min is adequately accomplished by the establishment of support equal to 25% of the cardiac output. This may be achieved with most forms of VA, VV, or arteriovenous ECMO.
4. Normal cardiac perfusion is maintained since the right atrium and ventricle are not decompressed, thus maintaining right and left coronary perfusion.
5. The patient must be able to achieve adequate cardiac function.
6. The arterial oxygenation ranges from 45-80 torr, which may be a consideration in patients with increased oxygen consumption.
7. The increased bypass flow to the right heart may increase lung volume and lead to pulmonary congestion.
8. Systemic circulation may need to be supported chemically.

Arteriovenous ECMO

Research has begun to show the adaptability of the cardiorespiratory system. Providing extracorporeal gas exchange without the use of a pump has been published.[27] Relying on the native cardiac output and access from a central artery through an extracorporeal circuit, the blood is returned to a central vein. This has been shown to provide adequate carbon dioxide removal in healthy subjects.[27] This technology is also capable of providing up to 50 mL/min of oxygen delivery.[27] The hurdle for endogenous cardiac support is the acquired increased myocardial oxygen consumption from the arteriovenous shunt and the need for increased oxygen delivery during illness. This has limited this application.

Artificial Placenta

Exploration of perinatal and fetal physiology has shed light on the application of ECLS. Normal intrauterine physiology supports fetal well-being with a unique range of parameters. Uterine implantation occurs at a pO_2 of approximately 15mmHg. This is believed to allow the fetus to develop at a low level of metabolism and therefore reduce the production of reactive oxygen species and oxidative stress.[28] The maternal circulation to the placenta is not fully established until the end of the first trimester.[28] Normal near-term placental oxygenation saturation is approximately 80%. Normal umbilical vein saturation is 70%. The high oxygen affinity and oxygen capacity of fetal blood provides umbilical venous blood with oxygen content of 6.6 mM.[29, 30, 31, 32, 33] This content is comparable to an adult arterial blood value. Normal fetal arterial saturations are then in the range of 40%. Fetal cerebral oxygen delivery occurs at a saturation of approximately 68%, and systemic oxygen delivery occurs at approximately 61% saturation. Total fetal cardiac output is approximately 500cc/kg/min.[28, 29, 30] Fetal oxygen consumption is calculated to be approximately 300 cc/min.[30, 31, 32] This is accomplished with fetal hemoglobin that allows oxygen delivery and extraction to occur at lower levels of saturation.

The term *fetus* is sustained with an arterial pH of 7.38. The result is that intrauterine physiology is capable of sustaining comparable resting adult oxygen consumption with an oxygen delivery at significantly lower saturation, while fetal distress has been noted to be clinically relevant when the venous saturation falls below 30% and the pH below 7.1, investigators have begun to look for the wider application of ECLS for newborns.[27, 31, 32, 33, 34]

The concept of an artificial placenta is to mimic the physiologic milieu of the infant. Access is gained from the arterial system and returned to the venous system. An extracorporeal pump or no pump may be utilized. A circuit volume equal to the infant volume is created to reduce extracorporeal capacity. A very low resistance circuit maximizes extracorporeal circulation and reduces extracorporeal cardiac load. Effective nonpump circulation for carbon dioxide has been achieved equal to 25% of native cardiac output, with no deleterious effects.[27, 32, 35] This is adequate for carbon dioxide removal with no deleterious cardiac effects to a normal newborn heart. Oxygen delivery of 2cc/kg/min has also been achieved.[27, 32, 35] This can prove to be inadequate if the physiologic demands are increased. The further advancement of low resistance, high-efficiency membranes, biocompatible circuits, low-resistance catheters, and newborn extracorporeal environmental systems will be forthcoming.[36, 37, 38] The scaling of these devices to treat all forms of respiratory failure in pediatric and adult intensive care units is imminent. Further advancements in the development of the extra uterine environment to mimic the additional functions of the umbilical circulation and the amniotic sac and its physiologic function are also serious considerations for the successful application of the concept.

Indications and Criteria

ECMO should be considered in any patient with acute, severe, reversible respiratory, cardiac, or cardiorespiratory failure after the unsuccessful applications of maximum medical management. The widespread use of high-frequency ventilation, nitric oxide, and surfactant has improved the care for countless children. This technology may improve or stabilize a patient but has also closed the safety time margin for many infants who do not respond or deteriorate. This places a strong need for improved communication between ECMO centers and referral centers. Regional ECMO centers have reported 10%-18% hidden mortality of interhospital transport deaths of ECMO candidates.[39, 40] ECMO reached a peak of clinical application in 1991 with over 1,500 cases reported to the ELSO registry for neonatal respiratory conditions with a current reported rate of approximately five hundred over the past six years.[22] This reflects recent advances in technology and perhaps the more judicious application of heroic therapy.

The most common indication for newborn infants is support in the treatment of congenital heart disease. Preop and postop cardiac surgery bridging as become an accepted resource of the newborn. Acute respiratory failure of less than fourteen days duration with maximum medical and ventilatory support is the next most common indication. The etiology may be derived from intrauterine hypoxia such as meconium aspiration, infection, delivery, or congenital abnormality such as congenital diaphragmatic hernia (CDH).

Published inclusion and exclusion criteria that have shown the best outcomes are shown below.[40, 22, 41, 42, 43, 44]

The acute presentation of any condition may obscure the reversibility and survivability to the family and caregivers. The ECMO team should make a clinical decision whether to proceed with ECMO based on the patient's history, physiologic instability, overall clinical condition, and estimated prognosis with and without ECMO, with consent of the family. The future availability, resources, and response time of the ECMO team—including ECMO specialists, operating room staff, and pediatric surgical team—should be taken into account realistically if cannulation is postponed. The entire ECMO team and family should clarify the patient's diagnosis and prognosis before the initiation of ECMO. The ECMO team must ensure that the family understands that not all children are able to reverse their disease process. ECMO is not designed to be used indefinitely or to prolong an inevitable death. The ECMO team's opportunity, within reasonable medical certainty, is to offer an acceptable quality of life and/or survival expectancy for at least one year. This discussion must be explored before ECMO has begun and then placed within the hands of the ECMO team after appropriate communication with the family.

General Newborn Inclusion Criteria and Exclusion Criteria[43,44]

- Gestational age ≥ 34 weeks and/or birth weight ≥ 2,000 grams.[*]
- No more than 10-14 days of assisted ventilation.[†]
- No significant intracranial hemorrhage (ICH), grade III or IV.[‡]
- No significant unrepairable cardiac or congenital abnormality.
- No lethal congenital abnormality.[§]
- No evidence of significant irreversible brain damage.
- Pulmonary physiologic maturation for CDH.[¶]
- No prolonged cardiac arrest.
- Uncontrolled hemorrhage may be a contraindication.
- Failure of maximum medical and ventilation management.[**]

---

[*] Unpublished data has improved survival for younger and smaller neonates

[†] Mechanical support of FiO_2 ≥ 0.65, PIP ≥ 35, PEEP ≥ 10, myocardial support with two or more inotropes

[‡] Grade II ICH is considered a relative contraindication

[§] Lethal trisomy expression is most common

[¶] CDH with one preductal blood gas values of saturation ≥ 90% and $PaCO_2$ ≤ 50 mmHg

[**] All measurements are relative to atmospheric conditions at sea level

As measured by

- Oxygenation Index ≥ 40 for four hours.[††]
- AaDO$_2$ ≥ 605 for four hours (sea level).[‡‡]
- PaO$_2$ ≤ 35 for four hours.
- Acidosis ≤ 7.25 for four hours.
- Ejection fraction ≤ 22%.
- Oxygenation index ≥ 25 is considered a candidate for transport to an ECMO center on maximum support.
- Oxygenation index of ≥ 45 is often used for infants on high-frequency ventilation.
- CDH indications include permissive hypercapnia and pH ≤ 7.15.

General Pediatric Inclusion and Exclusion Criteria

ECMO should be considered in any patient with acute, severe, reversible respiratory, cardiac, or cardiorespiratory failure after the unsuccessful applications of maximum medical management (see above as for newborns).

The duration and definition of significant ventilation varies from center to center, but below are some general pediatric guidelines. Most centers may agree that a PEEP greater than 15 cm H$_2$O, a mean airway pressure (MAP) greater than 25 cm H$_2$O, and a peak inspiratory pressure greater than 45 cm H$_2$O may induce injury if applied for many days.

OI greater than 40 for more than six hours while on a ventilator from twelve hours to seven days has been suggested to predict a 70% predicted.

Ventilator Days

< 2 years ≤ 10 days
2-8 years ≤ 8 days
> 8 years ≤ 6 days

[††] **OI** = $\dfrac{\text{mean airway pressure (MAP)} \times \text{FiO}_2 \times 100}{\text{PaO}_2 \text{ (postductal)}}$

[‡‡] **AaDO$_2$** = **a**lveolar **a**rterial **d**ifference **o**f **o**xygen (alveolar air equation)
    AaDO$_2$ = $((\text{FiO}_2(P_{atm} - P_{H2O})) - (\text{PaCO}_2 / \text{RQ}))$
    $- \text{PaO}_2$
This formula must be adjusted to the ambient altitude!

- A PaO$_2$/FiO$_2$ < 50 mmHg or a AaDO$_2$ > 600 mmHg may also suggest morbid respiratory failure.
- Patients with recalcitrant respiratory acidosis, pH < 7.15, and hypercapnia.
- A static lung compliance < 0.5 cc/cmHg$_2$O/kg.
- A persistent air leak syndrome should also be considered individually.
- Major hemorrhage or severe coagulopathy that may likely be uncontrollable on heparin.
- Life-threatening primary immunosuppression: previous solid organ transplant, previous bone marrow transplant, severe combined immune deficiency, or human immunodeficiency virus infection that is not treatable.
- Cardiac arrest with severe neurological impairment.
- Acute or chronic, severe central nervous system injury, including encephalitis, persistent vegetative state, encephalopathy, meningitis, or intractable seizures, and fixed and dilated pupils.
- Recent cerebral-vascular accident or severe traumatic brain injury.
- Severe, chronic lung disease requiring home ventilator dependence.
- Fixed elevated pulmonary vascular resistance.
- Lethal, terminal, and/or progressive congenital/genetic malformation(s), anatomic abnormalities, systemic, oncological, metabolic disease or major chromosomal abnormalities (trisomy 13, 18, etc.).

Congenital Diaphragmatic Hernia[43]

Criteria by failure to maintain with pre-ECMO therapy are the following:

- Preductal saturation ≥ 85%
- pH ≥ 7.25
- Gentle ventilation with pCO$_2$ ≥ 65-70
- Conventional: PIP ≤ 25, PEEP ≤ 10
- High frequency: MAP ≤ 20
- Common neonatal ECMO diagnosis[22]
- Perioperative cardiac surgery
- Persistent pulmonary hypertension with persistent fetal circulation
- Meconium aspiration
- Neonatal respiratory distress
- Sepsis
- Pneumonia
- Congenital diaphragmatic hernia
- Cardiomyopathy

Selected Pediatric ECMO Diagnosis

Common acute pediatric respiratory failure conditions:

- ARDS or acute hypoxemic respiratory failure
- Pneumonia (viral/bacteria/aspiration)
- Pulmonary embolus
- Posttraumatic
- Asthma or bronchiolitis (including secondary to RSV)
- Acute sickle-cell chest syndrome
- Near drowning
- Acute respiratory failure secondary to malignancy
- Cardiac diagnosis
- Preoperative and postoperative cardiac repair, postcardiac support
- Myocarditis
- Reversible cardiomyopathy
- Septic shock
- Pericardiac transplant (bridge to physiologic surgical correction)
- Cardiogenic shock including secondary to reversible toxic ingestions

Cardiac and Septic Shock ECMO Inclusion Criteria

- Acute, life-threatening, but potentially reversible cardiovascular decompensation that is unresponsive to maximum optimal medical management including, when appropriate, vasodilator and/or vasoconstrictive agents, inotropic agents, antiarrhythmic agents, and cardiac pacing
- Progressive hypotension < 2 SD for age
- LA or RA pressure greater than 20 mmHg for more than four hours
- Decreasing renal function oliguria: urine < 1 mL/kg/hr for two hours
- Tachyarrhythmias or bradyarrhythmias and/or low cardiac output secondary to reversible toxic drug effects
- Decreased SVO_2 < 60%
- Decreased systemic oxygenation; see also respiratory criteria above
- Persistent acidosis
- CI < 2.0 L/m^2
- Echocardiographic evidence of severe biventricular failure
- Ejection fraction < 22%
- Etiology of underlying heart disease and current decompensation known with reasonable degree of expectation for reversibility

Contraindications

- Ongoing cardiac arrest.
- Prolonged hypoxic ischemic insult.
- Prior cardiac arrest with unknown neurological status.
- Actual or possible major brain injury.
- Must be documented alert and responsive to verbal commands just prior to acute event or operation.
- Infants and children must be documented alert with reversal of paralysis and/or narcotics.
- Uncontrollable status epilepticus.
- Condition incompatible with normal healthy childhood.
- Prolonged period of shock more than twelve (12) hours.
- Uncontrolled septic shock will be assessed individually.
- Bleeding disorder will be assessed individually.

Special Considerations for the Pediatric ECMO Patient

The ELSO registry reports over five thousand pediatric respiratory cases with a 56% discharge rate. There are an equal number of pediatric cardiac cases with a reported survival rate of 48%.[22] This highlights the challenges of identifying reversible pediatric respiratory and cardiac disease. Placing a pediatric patient on ECMO for respiratory failure is a complex commitment. The approximate average length of ECMO for neonatal respiratory failure over the past five years is approximately 140 hours.[22] The pediatric respiratory failure ECMO run is over three hundred hours.[22] In general, the more sudden or acute the decompensation, the quicker the disease process may respond to appropriate therapy. The previously healthy pediatric patient placed on ECMO quickly for rapid deterioration may respond in a few days. The recovery is often within forty-eight to seventy-two hours, and weaning will proceed quickly, as seen in the newborn. If a child is placed on ECMO for a serious steady deterioration that has not responded to aggressive maximum therapy for several days, the course may be very protracted. It is not possible to give firm guidelines, and successful pediatric ECMO runs may last many weeks. The length of time on the pump should be continually assessed with the clinical condition of the child.

A long uncomplicated run with very slow but possible improvement is warranted. A long complicated run with progressive multiorgan failure over several weeks with no evidence of improvement is not appropriate. The ECMO team should realistically counsel the family regarding these possibilities prior to ECMO. The ECMO team's perception, and equally important the family's perception, of the condition of the child must be aligned initially and continuously. It is also very important to designate one individual to act as the communicator for these issues. Hearing several versions of this complex story will often confuse and hinder the best of intentions.

Adult Guidelines

- Reasonable likelihood of reversal of underlying disease.
- Control of the primary source of pulmonary failure.
- No secondary source of organ dysfunction.
- Reasonable cardiac ventricular function so that cardiac extracorporeal support is not necessary.
- Underlying disease with at least twelve months of expected survival.
- Clinical setting will tolerate anticoagulation.

Outcomes

The most common diagnosis reported to the ELSO registry in July 2011 are listed below.[22]

		Total	Survived ECLS	Survived D/C, transfer
Neonatal				
Respiratory		24,777	85%	75%
	MAS	7,814	94%	
	RDS	1,508	84%	
	PPHN/PFC	4,129	78%	
	CDH	6,280	51%	
Sepsis		2,626	75%	
Cardiac		4,375	61%	39%
ECPR		694	63%	39%
Pediatric				
Respiratory		5,009	65%	56%
Cardiac		5,423	64%	48%
ECPR		1,347	53%	40%
Adult				
Respiratory		2,620	63%	55%
Cardiac		1,680	53%	39%
ECPR		591	38%	29%

Complications

The most common complications encountered by newborns with respiratory Failure reported to the ELSO registry in July 2011, with an incidence of ≥ 10%, are listed below. (22)

Cardiovascular: inotropes on ECLS
20.1% of all patients:				61% survival
Mechanical: clots; oxygenator
17.2% of all patients:				65% survival
Mechanical: clots; bladder
15% of all patients:				68% survival
Renal: hemofiltration required
14.8% of all patients:				53% survival
Cardiovascular: hypertension requiring vasodilator
12.3% of all patients:				72% survival
Mechanical: cannula problems
11.7% of all patients:				67 % survival
Hemorrhagic: hemolysis
10.9% of all patients:				65% survival

Lethal Complications

Newborns with respiratory failure reported to the ELSO registry in July 2011 with a survival ≤ 40% are listed below.[22]

Neurologic: brain death clinically determined
0.9% of all patients:				0 % survival
Cardiovascular: tamponade; serious
0.2% of all patients:				35% survival
Renal: creatinine ≥ 3
1.4% of all patients:				36% survival
Metabolic: pH ≤ 7.20
3.3% of all patients:				38% survival
Hemorrhagic: disseminated intravascular coagulopathy (DIC)
2.5% of all patients:				39 % survival
Renal: dialysis required
3.2 % of all patients:				40 % survival

Physiology

Cardiopulmonary bypass is the maintenance of homeostasis when maximum medical therapy is inadequate. The goal is to assist native function by achieving adequate support for the patient's moment-to-moment metabolic demands. This requires an adequate assessment of endogenous pulmonary and/or cardiac function and the accurate understanding of the every changing balance between oxygen delivery and oxygen consumption. Initial support of the ECMO patient requires providing adequate exogenous oxygen delivery to allow the elimination or significant reduction of iatrogenic pulmonary injury. The time placed on exogenous support must rest the lungs and not contribute to further lung injury. The opportunity for recovery will depend upon adequate time for the pulmonary system to heal and renew adequate gas exchange. Exogenous cardiac support may also be required if the pathology has caused significant myocardial dysfunction, metabolic demands that cannot be met with endogenous cardiac output, or reversible perioperative cardiac depression.

Providing adequate ECMO support is primarily focused on the balance between oxygen delivery and oxygen consumption. Arteriovenous support supplies additional cardiac output. Oxygen delivery must be maintained at a level such that *adequate oxygen delivery* will be achieved for specific patient needs. These needs may change from time to time (such as sepsis and myocardial dysfunction). Complete oxygen delivery requirement for most patients at rest can be achieved with arteriovenous pump flows that deliver 80% of the predicted cardiac output. Cardiac output (CO) measurements in pediatrics is a complex target.[45,46,47,48] Newborn cardiac output measurements ranges from 120 to 200 mL/kg/min.[45,48] Doppler studies of left ventricular output have shown that the sick neonate may transiently increase output to 250 mL/kg/min.[45] The ECMO team will often use 120 mL/kg/min as the baseline newborn cardiac output. The ECMO team often uses 100 cc/kg/min for a child between two and eight years old and 80 cc/kg/min for pediatric patient eight to twelve years old as resting ECMO pump flow. The resting metabolic oxygen delivery requirement of neonates is approximately 6 cc/kg, children at 4-5 cc/kg, and adults at 3 cc/kg. Venovenous pump flows are indirectly related to oxygen delivery and will be discussed separately. The successful application of ECMO is dependent upon the thorough understanding of the factors that effect oxygenation and oxygen delivery. One must have a complete review of the concepts of arterial oxygen content (C_aO_2), venous oxygen content (C_vO_2), arteriovenous oxygen differences ($AVDO_2$), oxygen delivery (DO_2), oxygen consumption (VO_2), and oxygen extraction before applying ECMO to a patient. A thorough knowledge of oxygen-independent and oxygen-dependent physiology is also necessary. ECMO management requires the use of the following formulas.

Physiology Formulas

Oxygen Content = (mL O_2/100 mL blood, vol. %)

Total amount of oxygen (O_2) in the blood

- Arterial oxygen content = CaO_2
- Venous oxygen content = CvO_2
- CaO_2 = amount of O_2 bound to hemoglobin in the artery + amount of O_2 dissolved in the arterial blood
- CvO_2 = amount of O_2 bound to hemoglobin in the vein + amount of O_2 dissolved in the venous blood
- Amount of O_2 bound to Hgb = Hgb (gm/dl) × (% sat of Hgb) (1.36 mL O_2/gm. Hgb)
- Amount of O_2 dissolved in arterial blood = partial pressure of O_2 (paO_2)(torr) × (0.0031 mL O_2/dl/mmHg)
- Amount of O_2 dissolved in venous blood = partial pressure of O_2 (pvO_2) (torr) × (0.0031 mL O_2/dl/mmHg)

Example:

CaO_2 = ((Hgb) × (arterial sat) × (1.36)) + ((0.0031) × (paO_2))
Hgb = 12.0, sat = 100%, paO_2 = 100
CaO_2 = (12 × 1.0 × 1.36) + (0.0031 × 100)
CaO_2 = 16.63 vol %

CvO_2 = ((Hgb) × (mixed venous sat) × (1.36)) + ((0.0031) × (pvO_2))
Hgb = 12.0, sat = 70%, pvO_2 = 40
CvO_2 = (12 × 0.7 × 1.36) + (0.0031 × 40)
CvO_2 = 11.55 vol %

Arteriovenous Oxygen Difference

($AVDO_2$) (vol. %) = Oxygen Extraction

Difference in content between arterial oxygen content and venous oxygen content

$AVDO_2 = CaO_2 - CvO_2$
CaO_2 = 16.63 vol%, Hgb = 12.0, sat = 100%, paO_2 = 100
CvO_2 = 11.55 vol%, Hgb = 12.0, sat = 70%, pvO_2 = 40
Example above $AVDO_2 = CaO_2 - CvO_2$ = 16.63-11.55 = 5.12 vol %

Factors that Affect Oxygen Content

Example

Typical	*Arterial*	*Venous*
Hgb (gm/dl)	16	16
pO_2	100	40
%Sat (Hgb)	99%	75%
Oxygen Content	21.5	16.3

$AVDO_2 = CaO_2 - CvO_2$ = 21.5-16.3 = 5.2 vol %

Examples

PO_2 (mmHg)	Saturation (%0	Oxygen Content (vol. %)
600	100	22.5
100	100	20
75	95	19
55	87	18
40	75	15.5

Hemoglobin

Adult Hemoglobin Oxygen Disassociation Curve

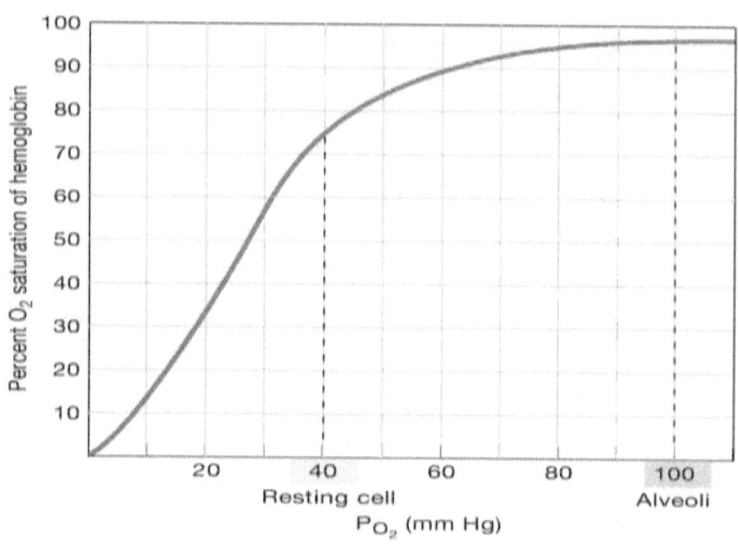

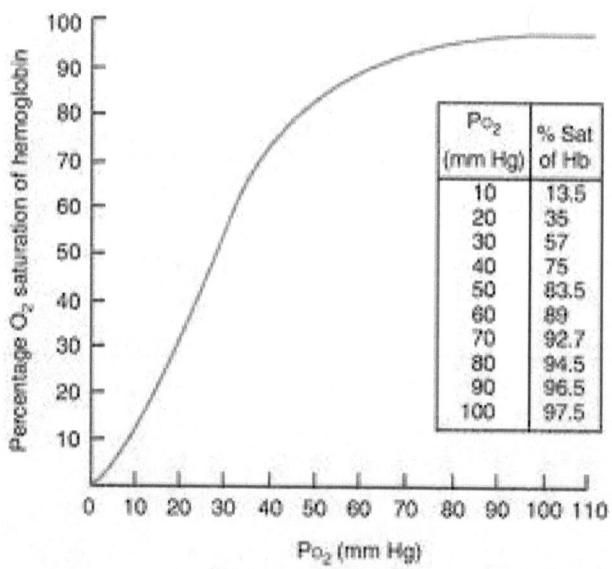

Physiologic oxygen content and physiologic oxygen extraction occurs within the normal hemoglobin oxygen disassociation curve

Factors that affect Hgb / O2 Disassociation Curve

Allosteric: Fetal, adult, hemoglobinopathy

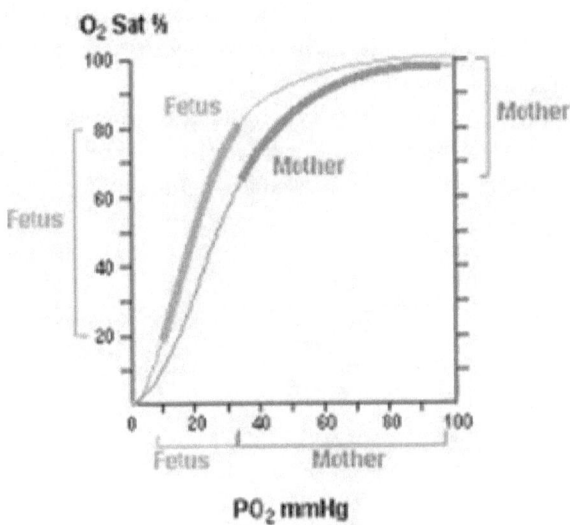

Fetal hemoglobin compared to adult hemoglobin

- **Adult Hemoglobin = HgA = $\alpha 2, \beta 2$ (90%), $HgA_2 = \alpha 2, \delta 2$ (10%).**
- **Fetal Hemoglobin = HgF = $\alpha 2, \gamma 2$ (80%), HgA / HgA_2 = 20%.**
- The different alpha and gamma chains create an allosteric difference of HgF to HgA or HgA_2.
- The allosteric change increases the affinity of fetal hemoglobin for oxygen compared to adult hemoglobin.
- Fetal hemoglobin also has a lower concentration of 2.3 diphosphoglycerate (DPG) than adult hemoglobin.
- This *"shift to the left"* of the hemoglobin oxygen disassociation curve due to HgF and decreased 2.3 DPG represents an increased affinity of fetal hemoglobin for oxygen and creates a higher hemoglobin saturation at lower oxygen tensions.
- This favors the binding and delivery of more oxygen at the lower fetal oxygen tensions.

Factors That Affect Hgb / O_2 Disassociation Curve

pH

- Increased hydrogen ion concentration [H^+] lowers the pH.
- Lowering of the pH (acidosis), such as what occurs in the peripheral tissue and pathophysiologically, decreases the affinity of hemoglobin for oxygen.
- This *"shift to the right"* favors the release of oxygen in a high-oxygen delivery / low-oxygen tension environment that might be the result of a pathologic condition that causes acidosis (i.e., sepsis).

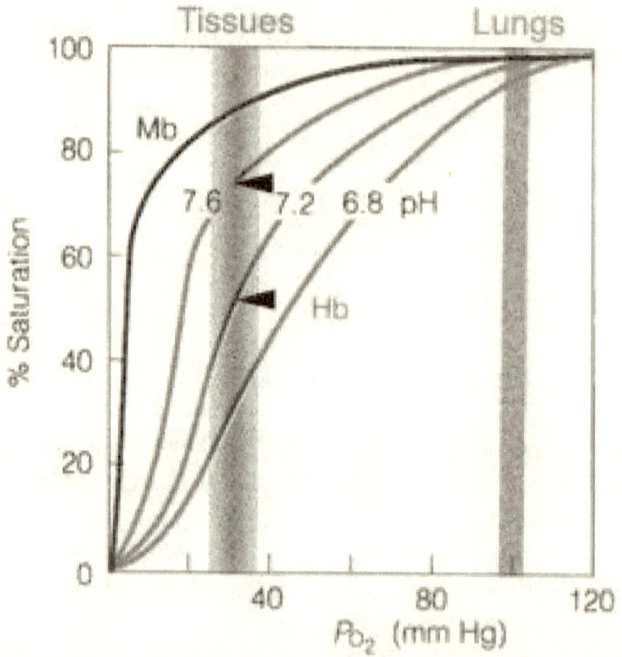

http://www.aw-bc.com/mathews/ch07/fi7p16.htm

Factors That Affect Hgb / O_2 Disassociation Curve

pCO_2

- **Increased carbon dioxide concentration [pCO_2] lowers the pH.**
- **Bohr effect is a direct effect on hemoglobin.**
- **Increased pCO_2 decreases the affinity of hemoglobin for oxygen.**

Temperature

Increased temperature decreases the affinity of hemoglobin for oxygen.

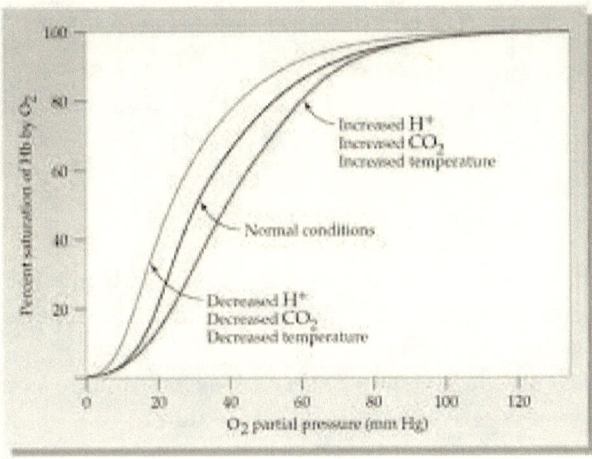

Factors That Affect Hgb / O_2 Disassociation Curve

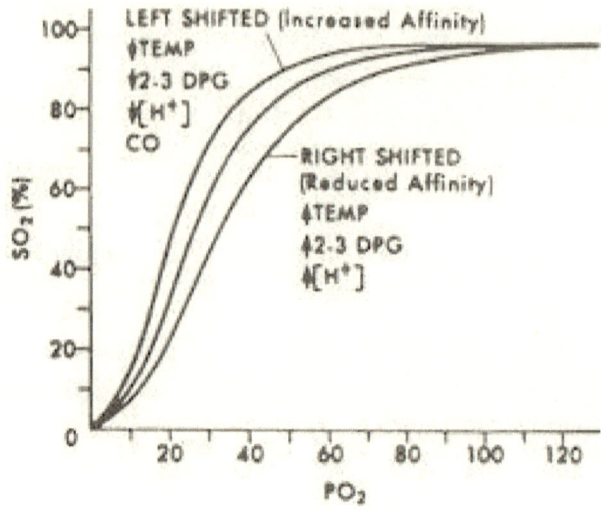

- A "shift to the right" represents a decreased affinity for Oxygen
- An increase in [H^+] acidosis, carbon dioxide, temperature, and 2.3 DPG reduces the affinity.
- This occurs during most stressed or pathologic conditions and improves oxygen delivery in a disease state.

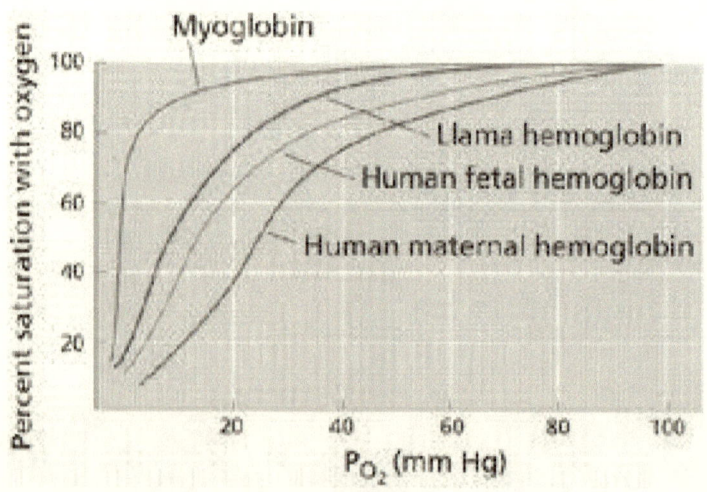

- A "shift to the left" represents an increased affinity for oxygen.
- A decrease in [H⁺] alkalosis, carbon dioxide, temperature, and 2.3 DPG increases the affinity.
- This occurs during physiologic low-oxygen tension environments such as in the fetus, myoglobin, and high-altitude environments.
- Oxygen delivery is improved in these physiologic conditions.

Oxygen Delivery = DO_2 = $Ca\ O_2$ × Total Flow

- $Ca\ O_2$ (oxygen content) = ((Hgb × arterial sat × 1.36)) + ((paO_2 × .0031)).
- Total flow = total natural (endogenous) corporeal flow (cardiac output (mL/min) + extracorporeal (exogenous) flow (mL/min).
- Total flow is equal to the cardiac output of the patient plus the extracorporeal pump flow.
- The extracorporeal flow is regulated during ECMO by increasing the amount of blood flowing through the ECMO pump. This extracorporeal flow is directly preload dependent and unloads the right atrium. Reduced flow from the right atrium will decrease the amount of blood flowing through the heart.
- Myocardial perfusion dependent upon intracardiac flow is decreased. The left ventricle is partially filled and thus has reduced left-ventricular output. Observing the arterial form tracing may represent the left-ventricular output.
- A calculation of the ratio of the systolic arterial pressure over the mean arterial pressure may roughly approximate left-ventricular output. The mean arterial pressure is managed to be normal within normal values for age.

Oxygen Delivery Theories

- **Total flow is directly proportional to oxygen delivery.**
- If endogenous cardiac output is fixed, then *changes in extracorporeal flow will directly affect oxygen delivery.*
- If flow is fixed, then changes in oxygen content will directly affect oxygen delivery.
- Oxygen delivery is directly proportional to ECMO flow.
- Oxygen delivery is directly proportional to oxygen content.
- If flow is fixed, then delivery is content dependent.
- If content is fixed, then delivery is flow dependent.

Factors That Affect Oxygen Delivery

Oxygen Content

Amount of Hemoglobin

$CaO_2 = ((Hgb) \times (art.\ sat.) \times (1.36)) + ((0.0031) \times (paO_2))$
$Hgb = 12.0$, $sat = 100\%$, $paO_2 = 100$
$CaO_2 = (12 \times 1.0 \times 1.36) + (0.0031 \times 100)$
$CaO_2 = 16.63$ vol %
$Hgb = 10.8$, $sat = 100\%$, $paO_2 = 100$
$CaO_2 = (10.8 \times 1.0 \times 1.36) + (0.0031 \times 100)$
$CaO_2 = 15$ vol %
$16.63/15 = 90\%$

A 10% change in Hgb causes a 10% change in oxygen content.

Factors that affect Oxygen Delivery

Oxygen Content
Hemoglobin saturation

$Hgb = 12.0$, $sat = 100\%$, $paO_2 = 100$
$CaO_2 = (12 \times 1.0 \times 1.36) + (0.0031 \times 100)$
$CaO_2 = 16.63$ vol %
$Hgb = 12.0$, $sat = 90\%$, $paO_2 = 100$
$CaO_2 = (12 \times 0.9 \times 1.36) + (0.0031 \times 100)$
$CaO_2 = 15$ vol %

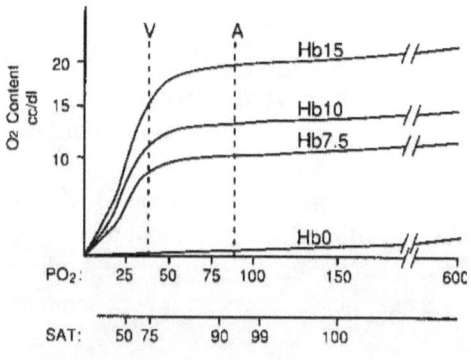

A 10% change in Hgb saturation causes a 10% change in oxygen content.

The three most important factors for oxygen delivery on ECMO are the following:

flow, hemoglobin, and saturation!

Other Factors Affecting Oxygen Delivery

- Type of hemoglobin
- Hemoglobinopathy
- Poisoning
- Native cardiac function (endogenous)
- Native cardiac anatomy
- Obstructive
- Shunts
- Restrictive cardiac pathophysiology
- Absolute extracorporeal flow (exogenous)
- Extracorporeal membrane factors
- Concentration of oxygen delivered
- Circuit malfunction
- Leak, obstruction, open clamp
- Inadequate flow
- Occlusion, obstruction, malfunction
- Membrane design
- Membrane flow rating
- Membrane surface area

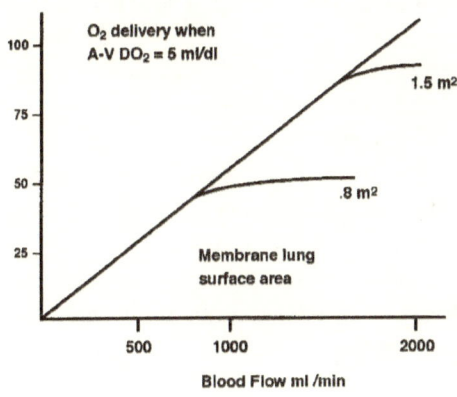

SciMed silicone membrane

- Quadrox hollow-fiber oxygenator.
- Pediatric Quadrox is rated 200cc/min-3.5 L/min.
- Newborn cardiac output is 100-300 cc/min.
- Quadrox D is rated from 500 cc/min up to 7 L/min.
- Pediatric cardiac output is 4-5 L/min (up to 45-kg child).
- Native pulmonary function.
- Endogenous shunts.
- Assisted Ventilation Factors.
- FiO_2 mean airway pressure.

Oxygen Consumption

Fick Principle

Adolf Eugene Fick (1829-1901) is credited with writing one of the first textbooks of biophysics in 1856.[34] Fick adapted the first law of thermodynamics, the conservation of energy and matter, when he stated that the flow through an organ (in his example, the body) is proportional to the amount of substrate entering and leaving the organ. A closed system and flow are taken as constants. The physiologic corollary states that if the total flow of the patient is constant, the oxygen delivery is constant, and all the variables relating to oxygen content are constant then; the oxygen extraction is a direct measurement of the oxygen consumed. Changes in oxygen extraction are changes in oxygen consumption.

The formula to represent the Fick principle in ECMO is found below:

Oxygen Consumption (VO_2) is directly proportional to ($\approx$) Flow × $AVDO_2$

- Flow = endogenous flow + exogenous flow.
- Endogenous and exogenous flow are constant.
- **$AVDO_2 \approx CaO_2 - CvO_2$**
- $CaO_2 = ((Hgb) \times (arterial\ sat) \times (1.34)) + ((0.0031) \times (paO_2))$.
- $CvO_2 = ((Hgb) \times (mixed\ venous\ sat) \times (1.34)) + ((0.0031) \times (pvO_2))$.
- Constants = Hgb, arterial saturation, 1.34, 0.0031, paO_2, pvO_2

- *Mixed venous saturation is the only variable.*
  Oxygen Consumption (VO_2) $\approx$ Mixed Venous Saturation (MVO_2)

- *Mixed venous saturation $\approx$ metabolism.*

- *Mixed venous saturation (MVO2) is a direct and continuous measurement of metabolism and VO2.*

Factors That Affect Oxygen Consumption

Increase

Hyperthermia, hypothermia without paralysis, infection, seizures, Inc. catecholamines, medication, trauma, malignancy, hyperthyroidism

Decrease

Paralysis, sedation, hypothermia with paralysis, medication, hypothyroidism

Mixed venous saturation is the most accurate measurement for adjusting the amount of oxygen delivery necessary.

Decreased MVO_2 with constant OD_2 describes the following:

- Increased metabolism.
- Increased VO_2.
- Altered
  oxygen distribution
  oxygen diffusion
  oxygen hemoglobin affinity
  oxygen utilization
- Distributive shock may decrease oxygen extraction during an increased metabolic state, resulting in an increased MVO_2.
- Increased MVO_2 in a sick patient may be sepsis.

Decreased MVO_2 requires increases in OD_2.

The three most important factors on ECMO for OD_2 are the following:

flow—hemoglobin—saturation

Oxygen Independent Metabolism

Henry's law describes the concentration of a gas based on its solubility.

$C = \alpha P$

A normal oxygen partial pressure in the artery paO_2 = 100.

A normal oxygen partial pressure in the vein is 40 (75% saturation).

$\alpha = 1.39 \times 10^{-3}$

$Ca = 1.39 \times 10^{-3} \times 100 = 139 \; \mu M \quad Cv = 1.39 \times 10^{-3} \times 40 = 56 \; \mu M$

Cellular metabolism has been found to be almost independent of oxygen tension to values of 20 μM.[35]

Venous oxygen partial pressure of 40 = 75% saturation of adult hemoglobin.

Mixed venous hemoglobin saturation of 75% provides double the quantity of oxygen necessary in the plasma for oxygen-independent cellular respiration.

Oxygen Consumption (VO_2) and Mixed Venous Saturation (MVO_2)

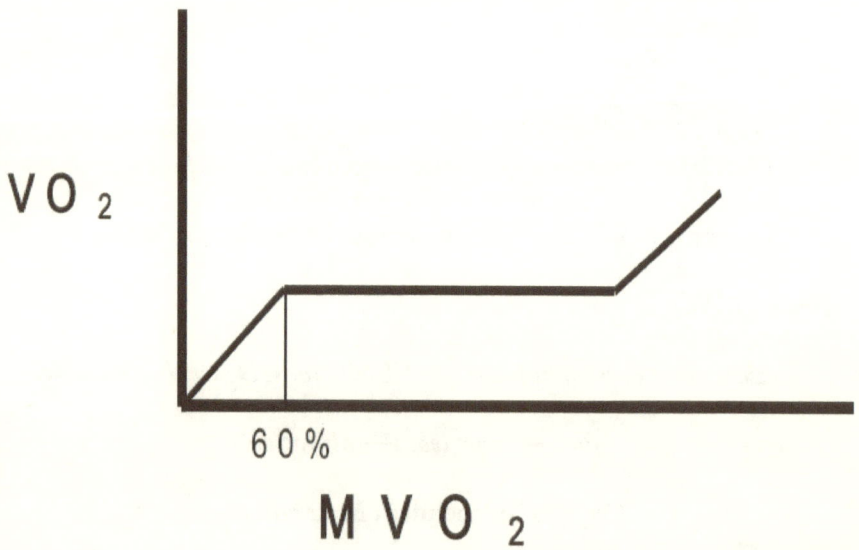

MVO$_2$ > 75% provides complete oxygen delivery for metabolic requirements

Exceptions: distributive shock, poisoning, metabolic derangement, malignancy, Hemoglobinopathy

Adequate oxygen delivery is confirmed by the absence of acidosis and increasing lactate levels.

Carbon Dioxide

The amount of CO$_2$ eliminated in extracorporeal circulation is a function of the membrane lung design, membrane material, membrane surface area, membrane ventilating gas flow (commonly called sweep flow), blood pvCO$_2$, and to a much lesser extent, blood flow. If the ventilating gas contains no carbon dioxide, the gradient for CO$_2$ transfer is the difference between the blood pvCO$_2$ and zero (when the gas flow rate is at or above the gas flow rate for the membrane). The pCO$_2$ drops during the passage of blood through the membrane lung, and the gradient decreases so that CO$_2$ excretion is less as the blood reaches the outlet. Consequently, the amount of CO$_2$ transfer is relatively independent of blood flow. The major determinant of carbon dioxide elimination is total surface area and flow rate of the sweep gas. The capacity for CO$_2$ removal is considerably greater than the capacity for oxygen uptake at the gas-rated flow. For all membrane oxygenators, CO$_2$ clearance will always be more efficient than oxygenation when the oxygenator is well ventilated and functioning properly. The extracorporeal membrane is generally *sized* to be capable of supplying total oxygen requirements. For this reason, the membrane lung will be capable of removing an excess of carbon dioxide. Extraneous CO$_2$ may be delivered in a combination gas (carbogen) with oxygen to the sweep gas in an effort to raise paCO$_2$.

If the native lung can supply some oxygenation and the intent of extracorporeal circulation is primarily CO$_2$ removal, this can be accomplished with endogenous venous access (VV ECMO) and relatively low blood flow. This is also known as ECCO$_2$R (pronounced "e-core") or extracorporeal CO$_2$ removal. There will be oxygenation provided by the membrane in both VV-ECMO and ECCO$_2$R, but no cardiovascular support and the oxygen delivery may be inadequate for physiologic requirements. The physiologic opportunity to improve venous pO$_2$ may provide increased oxygen delivery to the lungs, which may be the primary organ that is injured. The increase in venous saturation improves pulmonary *circulation by decreasing pulmonary hypoxia (pulmonary vasodilatation) and may lead to a secondary increase in arterial saturation.*

Hemodynamics

Factors That Affect ECMO Flow

ECMO flow is initially limited by the amount of venous blood drainage. This is dependent on the size, length, and position of the venous cannula and venous capacitance. Improper cannula placement and/or size will limit the ability to flow blood through the ECMO circuit. Decreased right-atrial filling will also decrease the ECMO flow.

The internal diameter and length of the venous drainage catheter and the internal diameter and length of the descending venous line to the bladder limit blood flow through the extracorporeal circuit. Resistance to blood flow varies directly with the length and diameter of the catheter. The capability of flow through the catheter is often referred to as the M number (Michigan), which is an empirical number derived from in vitro testing.[36] Consequently, the shortest and largest internal-diameter catheter that can be placed will allow the highest rate of extracorporeal blood flow. The superior vena cava allows the most direct access to the right atrium, and the right internal jugular vein usually has the largest diameter. A catheter placed through the right internal jugular vein into the atrium will usually permit venous drainage equivalent to the normal resting cardiac output of the patient. Blood drains via gravity from the right atrium. Many circuits use a reservoir to add capacitance to the circuit. This provides a volume differential to support more continuous flow. With or without a reservoir, the venous tubing enters a pump that provides the pressure to direct the blood through the membrane lung, heat exchanger, and back into the patient. There is significant resistance to flow through a silicone membrane lung and across the reinfusion catheter; therefore, the pressure on the arterial side of the circuit increases with increasing blood flow. In practice, a displacement pump is set to deliver the desired flow, and the postpump pressure is monitored. When using a silicone (Medtronic) oxygenator, postpressures as high as 300 mmHg are safe. Higher pressure may lead to a greater risk of blood leaks, hemolysis, or circuit disruption.

Commonly Used Single-Vessel Catheters[36]

Manufacturer	Size (F)	Flow (L) @ 100cm H_2O
Venous Catheter		
Biomedicus	8	0.5
	10	0.9
	12	1.5
	14	2.0
	19	2.6
	23	5.0
DLP		
	17	2.2
RMI	18	2.5
Arterial Catheters		
Biomedicus		
	8	0.5
	10	0.9
	12	1.5
	14	2.4
	21	5.0
	23	6.5
DPL		
	16	3.0

Microporous or hollow-fiber membranes are low-resistance oxygenators. This allows the nondiscriminatory use of nondisplacement (centrifugal) pumps. Low-resistance and nondisplacement devices eliminate the danger of increased circuit pressures. These low-resistance zero-pressure systems increase the safety of the circuit by eliminating the high pressure. The flow is completely dependent upon total absence of resistance. The presence of resistance in the venous catheter, circuit, arterial catheter, or the patient will reduce flow.

The vascular effect of venoarterial (VA) bypass on systemic perfusion is reflected in the arterial pulse contour and pulse pressure difference. Arterial pulse pressure and total blood flow vary during different levels of VA cardiopulmonary bypass. A patient on VA support may have adequate systemic blood flow with a flattened pulse contour. Extracorporeal blood flow during VA ECMO is initially maintained at approximately 80% of total predicted blood flow for the metabolic condition, and the newborn will have a pulse pressure of 10-15 mmHg.

Transient cardiac stun from the prime, acute increased aortic ECMO flow, myocardial dysfunction, electrolyte abnormalities, and acute reduced right atrial filling provide reversible conditions for the pulse contour to be flattened during early bypass.

The displaced extracorporeal pump creates a flow that is significantly less pulsatile. A nondisplacement pump is even less pulsatile, although some allow for a pulsatile alteration of flow. Arterial pulses may diminish when total bypass is reached. At total bypass, the left ventricle gradually fills with diminished pulmonary blood flow from the right atrium and bronchial and thesbian flow (flow directly from the coronaries back to the ventricle). This may lead to alteration of left ventricular end diastolic pressure and alterations of heart rate. In practice, it is unusual to completely unload the right atrium for any sustained period of time with extrathoracic cannulation as long as there is cardiac function. As long as oxygen delivery is adequate and native organ function is maintained, the presence of a pulse contour crucial.

The alteration of pulsatility may have an effect on flow-dependent organs such as the kidney. Fluctuations in flow will change the production of renin and catecholamines. The underlying changes in intravascular and extravascular volume and electrolyte changes during ECMO may also affect blood pressure. It appears that ECMO does cause an alteration of the usual response of the cerebral blood flow. Cerebral blood flow is pressure passive during the initiation of ECMO.[37] Risk factors for alterations in blood flow are related to the entire pre-ECMO condition, cannulation, and exposure to ECMO.

Blood Surface Interactions

ECMO requires continuous exposure of the entire blood volume to a large artificial surface. Protein and artificially coated surfaces reduce the blood component exposure to plasticizers, but red cells, white cells, platelets, and circulating protein molecules still come into contact with a foreign surface. This leads to an increase in inflammatory cytokines and compliment and neutrophil degranulation.[38, 39] In addition to the normal surface exposure, the flow patterns often include stagnant zones, eddy currents (back and forth), abrupt right-angle turns, rapid changes in velocity, compression, and the potential for jet and cavitation flow patterns. This increases the shear stress on blood components. Although the potential for damage to blood elements is great, hemolysis can be minimized and measured as serum-free hemoglobin or plasma Hgb. Platelets show the greatest effect of prolonged foreign-surface interaction. This is manifested by continuous platelet-aggregation formation and decreasing blood platelet count. Therefore, platelet levels must be kept greater than or equal to one hundred thousand. The acute massive hemodilution that occurs immediately upon the mixing during cannulation and insertion of bypass also causes a significant decrease in circulating platelets.

Chapter 2

Quality

Quality is the holy grail of any successful enterprise. Delivering superior quality is a prerequisite for success and has been directly linked to market share, return of investment, and cost reduction. [40, 41] The challenge to define, measure, improve, and control the quality of care provided in health care is paramount. Defining and measuring quality is one of the most important initial challenges facing health care. The ongoing goal is the continuous improvement of health-care services. Health care as a service industry may be described with two forms of quality: technical quality and functional quality.[42]

Technical Quality

We have published a reproducible and scalable measure of the technical quality for the highly complex process of therapeutic apheresis in the pediatric intensive care unit without additional capital cost.[43] The definition of quality we chose was obtained from the Donabedian theory of measuring the structure, process, and outcome.[44] We also referred to the Institute of Medicine definition of quality as "the degree in which health care services increases the likelihood of desired outcomes for individuals and population, and is consistent with current professional knowledge."[45] This incorporated two of Donabedain's three elements: measuring outcomes and assessing the adherence to processes that are proven while agreeing with patient preference or professional consensus (i.e., family directed care).[46]

Process / Six Sigma

The *process* is a collection of interacting components that transform inputs into outputs toward a common aim commonly called a mission statement.[47] Deming developed a famous systematic analysis and measurement of process for assessment of quality.[48] Following the contributions of Juran and Godfrey, this became know as total quality management (TQM).[49] A specific statistical technique of TQM known as Six Sigma is a tool to measure the distribution or variation of outputs in a process. Six Sigma measures the variation in a process. The goal is to achieve continuous improvement of the process, impact the outcome, and increase satisfaction.[47] A simplified but commonly utilized Six Sigma performance improvement model is the "*define, measure, analyze, improve, and control*" (DMAIC) model.[47] This step-by-step measurement tool evaluates a predefined process and quantifies whether the process is in control.[50]

The Institute of Medicine has reported a seminal finding that only 15% of medical errors are the result of inadequate individual performance, and the other 85% can be attributed to the system (structure) or processes.[45] Rubin described the advantages of measuring a process in health care and then comparing it to outcomes.[51] The advantages of measuring the process include providing feedback for quality improvement initiatives, it is less risky, and the data is quicker to collect. These investigators pointed out that there needs to be a strong relationship between the process and the outcome and that patient care is more about outcomes.[51] The disadvantage is that process measurement may be too specific and not reveal the comprehensive care. An Advisory Commission on Consumer Protection and Quality in the Health Care Industry, established in 1999, has recommended a strategic framework for a national quality measurement and reporting system.[52] This framework articulated the "criteria and process by which common measures should be selected, and to illustrate the results of applying this approach to one clinical area."[53] Quality improvement data has emerged with the use of these systems.[54]

Performance Improvement

We described the TA care as a step-by-step process. We designed a flowchart to carefully document each step of the process. We then defined each step with a unique clinical indictor (CI) that represented the exact task we felt provided quality care. A checklist was then created from this list of actions/goals.[55] The checklist was further refined to reflect finite collectable key clinical, operational, and patient/family data that the team established to reflect the directed values, events, and goals. This checklist was recorded real time during the care. This data was documented without the use of any patient-identifying information. This data was listed as clinical indicators (CI). The degree of compliance with these clinical indicators was analyzed and used as a metric for quality by calculating how close the process was running exactly as planned or "in control." We applied the theory of total quality management (TQM) through our "design, measure, analyze, improve, and control" (DMAIC) model. We were able to improve the process and bring it into control by increasing the compliance to more than 99% in the aggregate for the third and fourth quarters of the second year. Our publication documented technical quality by providing the desired outcome of our entire clinical process 99.75% of the time over the course of a year.[43]

The technical quality may be primarily defined by the accuracy of diagnosis, procedures, or outcomes.[43,56] This information is not generally available to the public, and what is available to the public may not be able to be adequately accessed and understood.[56] Functional quality refers to the manner in which service is delivered, and since patients may not be able to accurately assess technical quality, functional quality is usually the determinant of patients' quality perceptions. This also may be the most important variable influencing patients' value perception.[56]

Functional Quality

The challenges to measuring functional quality objectively have been described with three unique features: intangibility, heterogeneity, and inseparability of production and consumption.[41] The ability to measure intangible heterogeneic services when the production and consumption of that service cannot be separated leaves us with the choice to measure the perception of the services received. We are then left to measure perceived quality. Perceived quality is the consumer's judgment about overall excellence or superiority and results from a comparison of expectations with perceptions of performance.[57] Historically, the measure of quality has originated from the health-care provider and reported from their perception of technical quality. Combined with the fact that that patients are often unable to access and understand the technical quality of care, and we have a quality measurement challenge. Patients are now consumers who expect to receive the same service performance in health care as from other service industries and have unlimited access to information and choice. These consumers do not hesitate to change to an alternative health-care choice. This is why a service-marketing approach that looks at the recipient's perception is crucial.[57,58] The retention of customers by building brand loyalty has been shown to be five times less expensive that attracting new customers.[59]

Brand loyalty leads to the additional advantages of increasing referrals, increasing volume, and the opportunity for a pricing premium.[58] These are crucial for any successful business. The enhanced perception of quality also reduces the risk in providing the services and directly benefits the providers of the service.[58]

We then developed a project to measure the functional and perhaps superior measurement of quality for patients receiving TA.[41, 57] We chose the SERVQUAL method to measure functional quality. It is a measurement of the gap between the individual's expectations of service and the individual's perception of actual service provided.[41, 60]

SERVQUAL

SERVQUAL is an instrument developed with the support of the Marketing Science Institute. The purpose was to create a reliable, valid, and reproducible scale to assess customer perceptions of service quality across a broad range of services.[41] This scale relies on the definition of five dimensions of service critical to measuring customer perception.[41] The dimensions are the following: (1) tangibles like physical facilities, equipment, and appearance of personnel; (2) reliability, which is the ability to perform the promised services dependably and accurately; (3) responsiveness, the willingness to help customers and provide prompt service; (4) assurance, defined as the knowledge and courtesy of employees and their ability to inspire trust and confidence; and (5) empathy, which is caring, the individualized attention the firm provides its customers.[60]

These parameters are consistent with the work of Kohn in an Institute of Medicine report that defines patient-centered care as "care that is respectful of and responsive to individual patient preferences, needs, and values, and ensuring that patient values guide all clinical decisions."[61] Balint coined the term *patient center care*, and the Picker Institute, who outlined patient family directed care, defined the goal as dignity and respect, information sharing, participation and collaboration.[62] We have previously addressed the shortcomings of a technical measurement of quality and its correlation to quality.[43] The technical measurements to not alone address quality adequately to achieve the superior level of quality necessary to translate into measurable success in the health-care market. It is valid to identify patient/family perceptions and measure the gap between the patient/family expectations of service and the perception of quality service is delivered. Perhaps this is a truer measurement of quality.[41, 56, 63, 64, 65, 66, 67]

We found the functional quality measurements in the SERVQUAL survey more closely represented patient and family attitudes and perceptions and the actual perceived quality of the TA process (Sussmane J. unpublished data).

The undertaking of the provision of any extracorporeal life support technology is intellectually, financially, and technically complex. The burden to the health-care system, the patient and the families, is enormous. It is imperative that all providers are actively participating in the finest structure possible to ensure the highest levels of technical and functional quality. It is only through this rigorous pursuit of quality that we are able to deliver what we promise.

The following chapters regarding the precannulation, cannulation, and medical management of the patient is full of lists of activities.

A more complete guide to the fundamentals and practical application of quality in the PICU may be found in the *ECMO Study Guide: A Brief Practical Application of ECLS* (forthcoming) (Sussmane J., Xlibris).

It is strongly recommended that the* team *create active accurate process and use checklists to improve and maintain quality. [43, 55]

Chapter 3

Precannulation

Consent is a critical event for the family and the team. It is the crucial opportunity to establish the long-term successful relationship with the family. It is based on honest, direct, mutually meaningful communication. One member of the team must convey the thorough understanding that, in the team's opinion, this critical condition has not responded to maximum conventional medical treatment. It is often not possible to provide the family with a complete understanding of the condition, but they also must understand that in the opinion of the ECMO team, children who have not improved with the current treatment have a very small chance of surviving.

Extracorporeal membrane oxygenation (ECMO) must be provided based on the ECMO team's adherence to internal policies and procedures. An experienced center should provide the family with the confidence that the team is doing what it does best, and this is based on the individual center's experience.

The technique, application, and all procedures should be clearly described, with the team's reasonable expectations as to time required, personnel, equipment, potential benefits, sedation, pain, and complications. An open and frank discussion with the family about the expectations for length of time on bypass and recovery are also important. This should include a discussion about what the team will do if there is no recovery or life-limiting complications. Establishing the expectation that ECMO may not help and must be discontinued if it is not prolonging life, rather prolonging death, is best done precannulation.

Precannulation Evaluation

A high-quality quaternary referral center for ECMO places far fewer patients on bypass than referred. The results are often less than 30% of the children referred for ECMO are placed on bypass (Sussmane unpublished data). The explanation for this seemingly low number is the meticulous, thorough precannulation evaluation that must occur before cannulation.

- Complacency in accepting patient condition is not acceptable.
- Avoid cannulation and bypass emergencies.
- Avoid unnecessary and perhaps fatal bypass treatment.
- Avoid futile ECMO runs.

It is strongly recommended that the **team** *creates an accurate, complete, and active process of* **all** *activities to improve and maintain quality.*

- o **The patients' underlying condition must be confirmed to the highest degree of certainty.**
  - Full pre-ECMO evaluation must rule out correctable conditions.
    - Structural cardiac lesions
      - o Anomalous pulmonary venous return is still the most common correctable structural condition neonates are placed on ECMO.
    - Hemorrhage
      - o Intracranial
      - o Intrathorax
      - o Intra-abdominal
    - Pneumothorax
    - Genetic
    - Metabolic
    - Malignancy
    - Poisoning / toxin
    - Shock
      - o **Hypovolemic shock is the most common *correctable* presentation of the pre-ECMO neonate** (Sussmane unpublished data).
    - Iatrogenic
      - o Extubation, ventilator error, medication error

- o **Aggressive medical management must be propelled through the staff to the patient.**

    - Correction of iatrogenic conditions.
    - Volume resuscitation is crucial.
    - Correction of structural etiology.
    - Restoration of adequate hemoglobin.
    - Correction of iatrogenic conditions.

- o **The source of any immediate deterioration must be examined and treated.**

    - Completion of pre-ECMO orders are essential.
      - CXR, blood gas, H/H, platelets, cardiac ECHO, and cranial ultrasound are the minimal requirements.

Performance Improvement

It is strongly recommended that the *team* creates an accurate, complete, and active process of *all* activities to improve and maintain quality.

Precannulation Process

Once the decision has been made that a patient meets ECMO criteria, certain pre-ECMO procedures must be completed.

The PICU intensivist must be consulted. A consult or progress note must be written by the PICU fellow. This note must include all pertinent ELSO registry data:

a. Age
b. Weight
c. Height
d. Head circumference
c. Diagnosis (primary and secondary)
d. Length of ventilation
e. Ventilator settings, including MAP and inspiratory time
f. last ABG preductal and postductal
g. Acute criteria

1. $AaDO_2$
2. Oxygenation index
3. Acute deterioration of pO_2, pCO_2, and pH
4. Barotrauma
5. Cardiac arrest

1. The ECMO director and clinical coordinator must be notified of the consult and/or impending ECMO.
2. The surgical director of ECMO will be notified as soon as a consult or impending ECMO has been identified.
3. The attending ECMO physician or designee will order the following as STAT.

Pre-ECMO Orders

1. Type and crossmatch for the following: **STAT.**
2. Four (4) units PRBCs to include one (1) quad packed, leuko-reduced; two (2) washed units, one (1) for the pump and one (1) for the patient; two (2) units on hold in blood bank. For neonates, all blood must be washed, irradiated, and CMV negative.
3. One (1) unit FFP (fresh frozen plasma).
4. Two (2) units single donor platelets on hold.
5. Brain ultrasound stat to rule out intraventricular hemorrhage.
6. Echocardiogram stat to rule out cardiac malformations.
7. Laboratory studies: STAT

    a. CBC with differential
    b. Platelet count
    c. Fibrinogen
    d. Fibrin split products
    e. ACT stat
    f. P8, Ca^{++}, Mg^{++}

8. Central venous access to monitor CVP.
9. Urinary catheter.
10. Naso or oral gastric tube to gravity.
11. The following parameters should be corrected:

    a. Platelet count > 100,000; if not, transfuse one superpack platelets
    b. HGB/HCT > 15/45; if not, transfuse 10 mL/kg PRBCs

c. PT/PTT < 13/45
   d. PT > 13, give 1 mg Vitamin K stat
   e. PTT > 45, give 10 mL/kg FFP stat

12. Surgical area: the critical care unit needs to be prepared as for a cannulation procedure. Strict sterile technique should be employed.
13. The consent must be obtained prior to the procedure unless it is emergent.
14. Provide family with ECMO pamphlet and brochure and information folder.

Blood Bank Protocol

When the ECMO physician activates the ECMO team, it is the duty of the PICU charge nurse to notify the blood bank of the blood products required. The PICU charge nurse must ensure that the blood is drawn immediately upon the patient's arrival and that someone is specifically designated to transport the blood directly to the blood bank for processing. The patient must be immediately typed and crossmatched for the following:

All Blood Bank Orders Are STAT

1. Four (4) units washed PRBCs, one (1) quadpacked, one (1) washed, two (2) on hold at all times
2. One (1) unit of fresh frozen plasma (FFP)
3. Two (2) units single-donor platelets (on hold)
1. One (1) unit washed PRBCs

If patient condition deteriorates, physician may be required to order emergency typed but not crossmatched blood.

It is the responsibility of the blood bank to inform the PICU charge nurse that the blood has been processed. It is the responsibility of the PICU charge nurse and ECMO specialist to follow up on the blood processing and have the blood sent up to the PICU immediately after processing. Blood not required for immediate use should be placed in the PICU blood refrigerator.

In the instance of refrigerator failure, all blood products must be stored in the recovery room blood refrigerator. The temperature must continue to be monitored as stated above. If the recovery room refrigerator is not available, all blood products must be stored in the main blood bank.

Once the ECMO case is completed, all blood products must be returned to the main blood bank. This is the responsibility of the decannulating ECMO specialist.

ECMO Specialist Responsibilities Prebypass

1. Gather equipment

    a. ECMO cart (neonatal / pediatric)
    b. Infusion pump (micro)
    c. Extension cords (2)
    d. Transonic flowmeter and probe
    e. ECMO pump / stand / battery / heat exchanger
    f. ACT device (Istat, Hemochron)
    g. Better bladder reservoir and holder
    h. Platforms
    i. SvO2 computer (CDI)
    j. Needle box
    k. ECMO warmer bed
    l. Autosyringe
    m. I-Stat ACT cartridges
    n. Gas blender
    o. ECMO tubing pack (size dependent)
    p. Oxygenator (size dependent)
    q. Heat exchanger (if necessary)
    r. Arterial and venous cannulas (size dependent)
    s. Double-lumen venous cannulas (if requested)
    t. Tubing clamps (10)
    a. Flow cartridges if necessary
    b. Stopcocks
    c. Sterile gloves (size dependent)
    d. Chux pads
    e. Sharps disposal container
    f. Masks
    g. Surgical caps
    h. Tie gun and tie bands

2. The following disposables are to be collected from PICU supply and must be charged to the patient:

a. Priming set
   b. Microcassettes
   c. Package three-by-three nonsterile gauze
   d. Pressure monitoring IV set

3. The following medications are obtained from pharmacy stock:

   a. $D_{10}W$ 500 mL.
   b. Albumin 25% 50 mL.
   c. Sodium bicarbonate 8.4% 20 mL.
   d. Albumin 5% 100 mL.
   e. Calcium chloride
   f. Heparin (will need to be ordered from the pharmacy)

4. Check blood for newborns < 3.5 kg; larger infants, pediatrics, and adults need more.

   a. 2 units PRBCs (1 quad)
   b. 1 unit FFP
   c. 2 units platelets (on hold)

5. Send pre-ECMO orders to pharmacy for heparin bolus and drip.
6. Calibrate SvO_2 monitor.
7. Set up pressure monitor.
8. Cannulae sizes:

   a. Give scrub personnel the cannulas per surgeon preference.
   b. Sizes vary based on patient size, with vessel size and surgeon preference.

9. A prebolus patient ACT is performed. Also, once the blood prime is complete, a prebypass ACT from the pump is done.
10. The ECMO specialist is responsible for documenting the complete priming procedure.
11. Miscellaneous

   - Assist perfusionist with caps, tie bands, etc.
   - Document procedure, pre-ECMO vitals, ventilator settings
   - Prepare saline flushes
   - Draw up blood products
   - Notify "ECMO moms and dads" support group

Additional Safety Checklist

1. Plug in all equipment.
2. Do not use extension cords on the pump or heater.
3. Place the pump on the opposite side of the bed from the ventilator.
4. Check safety of water and preheat water heater.
5. Check the pump foreign objects

    II. If using a roller pump, check that the guides and rollers turn freely and are free of nicks.
    III. Be sure there are two tubing guides and one hand crank.

6. Turn on the pump and calibrate pump to proper tubing size used if necessary.
7. Check the blender per protocol.
8. Turn on the heater, set the temperature to 38°C, and check the water temperature in a few minutes. Check that the water level is just to the bottom of the screen. **Use sterile water only.**
9. Turn on the CDI monitor and allow it to warm up.
10. Complete the quality control for ACT device per protocol.

Circuit Priming Process

The following should be used as a guide for the purposes of setting up the circuit for ECMO for respiratory failure. This guide will assist with choosing the correct oxygenator, tubing pack, and cannulas for neck cannulation based on the patient size as determined by the weight in kilograms.

Weight (kg)	3-8 kg	9-14 kg	15-30 kg	30-55 kg	> 55 kg
Tubing Pack	Neonatal 1/4"	Neonatal 1/4"	Pediatric 3/8"	Adult 3/8"	Adult 3/8"
Raceway Size (occlusion pump)	1/4"	3/8"	3/8"	1/2"	1/2"
Oxygenator (**Quadrox**)	Mini	Pediatric	Pediatric	Adult	Adult

Oxygenator (Medtronics)	0800	1500	2500	3500	4500
Max. Flow	500 mL-1 L/min.	900 mL-1,500 mL/min.	1.5 L/min.-4.5 L/min.	2.8 L/min.-5.5 L/min.	5.5 L/min.-6.5 L/min.
Venous Cannula	10,12,14 Fr.	12,14 Fr.	12,14 Fr.	14,18,20 Fr.	20,24 Fr.
Arterial Cannula	8,10,12 Fr.	10,12,14 Fr.	12,14 Fr.	14,16 Fr.	14,16 Fr.
Required units of PRBCs	1 unit	2 units	2 units	2-3 units	3 units

ECMO patients who have a higher metabolic demand such as sepsis, shock, multiorgan dysfunction, or require increased oxygen delivery during VV-ECMO may require an oxygenator one size larger than indicated on this chart. Percutaneuos femoral cannulas may be required for increased venous return and in larger patients.

Circuit Setup

CIRCUIT SETUP

Medtronic Oxygenator / Cobe Occulsion Pump / Better Bladder / Transonic Flowmeter

1. Gather equipment: pump with stand, heat exchanger, blender, clamps, tubing pack, appropriate-sized oxygenator, infusion pumps, CDI monitor, Transonic flowmeter, and probe.
2. Check package integrity of ECMO tubing pack and oxygenator for physical defects such as cracked ports, damaged wrap, and patent O_2 ports.
3. Check that pump and electronics are working.
4. Make sure appropriate-sized tubing inserts are in the raceway (black = 1/4", white = 3/8", gray = 1/2").
5. Remove the heat exchanger and place in the bracket with the blood inlet on top and water connections facing away from the pump. Place pigtails on top of heat exchanger, making sure stopcocks are closed.
6. Hang Plasmalyte on pump IV pole.

7. Don proper personal protection equipment (PPE), including surgical hat, mask, and gloves when assembling sterile equipment and tubing pack.
8. Have someone open the Medtronic oxygenator box and place in the bracket with the blood outlet on the top (red capped). The writing on outside of oxygenator should be right-side up. Place pigtails top and bottom of oxygenator, making sure stopcocks are closed.
9. Have someone open sterile pack and place outer sterile wrap on the floor under the bladder box (to keep tubing that drapes on the floor sterile). Tighten all pigtails and stopcocks in the tray before removing any tubing.
10. Remove reservoir bag from tray. Hang bag from IV pole using a tubing clamp to hold yellow port top of bag. Clamp discard line and priming solution line (orange filter).
11. Connect venous tubing from bag (blue tape) to venous side of patient bypass bridge (blue tape). Connect arterial tubing from bag (red tape) to arterial side of patient bypass bridge (red tape).
12. Connect venous tubing coming down from patient bridge; place pigtails proximal to bladder box. Place bladder in bladder box and ensure there is no twisting of tubing.
13. Following lay of raceway tubing, place raceway tubing in tubing guides left first and then right; locking gates *do not* place tubing in raceway at this time. Blood path must be unobstructed for CO_2 flush and vacuum prime.
14. Connect tubing from raceway to port (remove blue cap) bottom of oxygenator.
15. Place eighteen-inch tubing with longer side to top of oxygenator (remove red cap); connect other end to top of heat exchanger.
16. Connect long arterial tubing from below arterial side of patient bridge to bottom of heat exchanger.
17. Heat exchanger water testing. Check for water cleanliness. Fill with distilled or sterile water to fill line (above mesh). Connect water lines to heat exchanger with water going in bottom and coming out top. Direction of water flow must be countercurrent to blood flow for optimal heat exchange. Open the valves and turn on the heater. Never restrict water outlet because it may overpressurize water path and cause water leak. Set heater temperature at 37.5°C. Test heat exchanger for water leaks for at least five minutes.

A dry, sterile, intact circuit may be usable for up to thirty (30) days.

CO_2 Prime

18. Place sterile green gas filter (in the pack) into the line and attach to 100% CO_2 tank (follow flow direction arrow on filter). CO_2 must be filtered with bacteriological filter since it is entering the blood path.
19. Place tubing clamp between upper and lower pigtails prebladder. Open one stopcock on pigtail proximal to clamp (closet to bridge). Place CO_2 line into stopcock on pigtail distal to clamp (before bladder) and open stopcock.
20. Place tubing clamps on patient bypass bridge and the prebypass filter line. Close the clamps on the prime bag discard line and blood prime line (orange filter).
21. Flowmeter on blender *must be off*.
22. Connect gas line green (¼" end) to oxygenator O_2 *inlet* on top of oxygenator. Connect vacuum line to oxygenator O_2 *outlet* (bottom of oxygenator) and clamp.
23. Slowly turn on CO_2 (0.2-0.5 L/min), watching prime bag for filling and listening for CO_2 release out of stopcock. Gas should be turned on just high enough to completely fill prime bag, and primer should be able to hear gas released through stopcock (max 7 L/min). Open clamps on two bypass lines for fifteen seconds to flush out air. CO_2 flush for at least five minutes. (CO_2 flush replaces air with CO_2, making debubbling easier during circuit priming. CO_2 provides a safety mechanism as it is more soluble in blood, so it would be less detrimental to patient in the event that a bubble remained in circuit).
24. Entire circuit must be closed (except one exit port on prebladder pigtail) for CO_2 to flush air through circuit. After five minutes, turn off CO_2, close CO_2 and release stopcock.
25. Remove clamp from vacuum line (oxygenator outlet) and turn vacuum up to 120-150 mm Hg. (vacuum source must not exceed—500 mmHg; membrane rupture may occur). Remove all clamps from circuit. Green tubing should be connected between O_2 inlet (top of oxygenator) and flowmeter. FLOWMETER SHOULD BE OFF. System should be totally closed; prime bag and bladder should collapse immediately if there is no leak in system. Leave vacuum on for at least five minutes.
26. Remove all open stopcock caps and replace with closed caps.

Save the package labels with the lot numbers and expiration dates of all items used. Store in the ECMO cart until the end of the case. Write the date and time the circuit was set up and CO_2 flushed.

Crystalloid Priming and Setting Occlusion

Crystalloid primed sterile circuit may remain intact for patient use for seven days.

1. Turn silence on (two outside switches circuit control box to up/on position—lights on) and override on (switch in center of circuit control box to on override/down position).
2. Clamp off all outlets from prime bag.
3. Clamp the AV bridge on the circuit and clamp the prebypass filter.
4. Spike the Plasmalyte bag and fill prime bag through blood filter (orange) line.
5. Debubble and bleed out air through stopcock on the top of prime bag.
6. Place clamp just distal to bladder, and clamp patient bypass bridge.
7. Open venous line slowly, "walking" fluid toward bladder. Remove air from bladder via stopcock on top of bladder.
8. Place a clamp on oxygenator inlet line between the oxygenator and pump roller head. Open stopcock on tubing proximal to oxygenator to air.
9. Swing both clamp gates out. Ensure that both tubing inserts are in place for proper-size tubing. Place tubing in raceway. Close clamp gates and adjust tubing retainers by using clamp adjustment knobs. (Retainers should be tight enough so that tubing cannot be pulled through.) Ensure that tubing is placed so that it rests evenly between the two roller guides.
10. Position rollers at nine o'clock and three o'clock and turn occlusion thumbwheel to completely occlude tubing.
11. Remove clamp between bladder box and roller pump. (Fluid level should not rise if tubing is occluded.) Very slowly move occlusion thumbwheel inward until fluid begins to rise at 1 cm/minute.
12. Move roller 180 degrees and position rollers at nine and three o'clock. Observe fluid moving at 1 cm/minute. Reset occlusion if necessary.
13. After occlusion set, close stopcock and remove tubing from roller head, leaving tubing in the inlet gate clamps.
14. Check heat exchanger for water leaks (check for moisture in tubing at blood outlet and water, check atmospheric vent).
15. Remove tubing clamp from oxygenator inlet, allowing rapid priming of oxygenator and heat exchanger.
16. Insert tubing into roller head by slowly advancing roller pump with hand crank while feeding tubing under/between roller guides following

natural bend of tubing. Leave enough tubing on negative side (bladder side) of roller pump to allow for future use ("walk the raceway").

17. Remove clamp on *arterial* inlet line on bag with prebypass filter.
18. Turn on pump and recirculate through AV loop.
19. Open bridge clamps to debubble bridges.
20. Open stopcocks to debubble pigtails and stopcocks.
21. *Gently* tap oxygenator to remove air using an open hand. Repeat as necessary.
22. Turn heat exchanger upside down and tap *gently* to remove air (do not strike the oxygenator or heat exchanger on end caps). Repeat as necessary.
23. Do not exceed 1 L/min flow during priming as a membrane shift could occur. After circuit is debubbled, remove vacuum from O_2 outlet.
24. Tie band all positive connections that are not bonded, including heat exchanger outlet. Before banding, be sure that tubing is on connectors as far as they will go.
25. To debubble bridge, turn off pump, unclamp the bridge, and send air up arterial line. Reclamp bridge.
26. Purge all pigtails. Note: when purging pigtails prebladder, the roller pump must be turned off to avoid negative pressure and air entering venous line.
27. Set up pressure monitors: preoxygenator, postoxygenator, bladder pressure.
28. Prime the pre and post oxygenator transducers with Plasmalyte.
29. Connect preoxygenator and postoxygenator transducers with an airless connection to the pigtails.
30. Connect the nonfluid-filled bladder pressure transducer connection to the bladder pressure monitor.
31. Connect pressure transducer cables to the appropriate transducers.
32. Zero each pressure transducer and set the high and low limits.
33. Document the date and time the circuit was crystalloid primed, along with all lot numbers and expiration dates.
34. Turn off the pump and remove all the clamps from the circuit if it is not going to be used immediately.

Blood Prime

Supplies Needed

- Neonatal circuit

    - Packed red blood cells (one [1] unit, washed)
    - Heparin (250 units)
        - 250 units = 1/4 mL of 1,000 u/mL
    - Sodium bicarbonate (8% NaHCO$_3$) (10 mEq)
        - 10 mEq = 10 mL
    - Fresh frozen plasma with filter (50 mL)
    - 25% albumin (50 mL)
    - Calcium chloride (10 % CaCl$_2$) (500 mg)
        - 500 mg = 5 mL of 100 mg/mL

- Pediatric / adult circuit

    - Packed red blood cells (one [1] unit, washed)
    - Heparin (500 units)
        - 500 units = 1/2 mL of 1,000 u/mL
    - Sodium bicarbonate (8% NaHCO$_3$) (20 mEq)
        - 20 mEq = 20 mL
    - Fresh frozen plasma with filter (100 mL)
    - 25% albumin (50 mL)
    - Calcium chloride (10% CaCl$_2$) (1,000 mg)
        - 1000 mg = 10 mL of 100 mg/mL

1. Turn off pump.
2. Turn on the heater and circulate with the temperature at 37°C.
3. Clamp two (2) outside tubes on prime bag (arterial and venous); leave middle Plasmalyte prime line open. (Note: clamp as close to bag as possible to save blood.)
4. Lower Plasmalyte bag, unclamp, and let prime bag drain into empty Plasmalyte bag.
5. Attach discard line (under prebypass filter) to patient port of a suction canister; leave tubing clamped (leave vacuum port on canister open to air).
6. Attach a 60 cc syringe to bladder stopcock and remove 50 mL of volume from bladder (to prevent dilution of prime); close stopcock.

7. Remove Plasmalyte bag and attach one (1) washed unit PRBCs with a blood filter. Open to prime bag and fill prime bag.
8. Make sure tubing from each side of prime bag remains clamped.
9. Have additional washed PRBC quad packs available on unit.
10. Prime venous side first (route of flow) by removing venous clamp closest to prime bag (note: when clamp opened, blood will gush and stop at bladder; this is normal).
11. Clamp venous tubing just before bladder and remove crystalloid from bladder with 60 mL syringe; close stopcock.
12. Unclamp venous line at bladder and discard line to suction canister.
13. Slowly turn on pump and start flow (approximately 25 mL/min); watch blood bag to prevent bag from emptying; observe waste line and increase flow until steady stream of prime enters the canister.
14. When blood reaches top of oxygenator, *turn off pump*.
15. Invert bladder.

16. **Add medications to bladder *in this order*.**

    a. Note: volume will increase backward into prime bag; that's okay.

    - Neonatal circuit

        - Heparin (250 units)
            - 250 units (1/4 mL of 1,000 u/mL)
        - Sodium bicarbonate (10 mEq of 8% $NaHCO_3$)
            - 10 mEq = 10 mL
        - 25 % albumin (50 mL)
        - Fresh frozen plasma with filter (50 mL)
        - Calcium chloride (10% $CaCl_2$) (500 mg)
            - 500 mg = 5 mL of 100 mg/mL

    - Pediatric / adult circuit

        - Heparin (500 units)
            - 500 units (1/2 mL of 1,000 u/mL)
        - Sodium bicarbonate (20 mEq of 8% $NaHCO_3$)
            - 20 mEq = 20 mL
        - 25 % albumin (50 mL)
        - Fresh frozen plasma with filter (100 mL)
        - Calcium chloride (10% $CaCl_2$) (1,000 mg)
            - 1,000 mg = 10 mL of 100 mg/mL

17. Turn off bladder stopcock.
18. Clamp arterial line just above the discard line and open discard line.
19. Turn on pump slowly, approximately 25 mL/min, until blood shows in discard line.
20. Watch priming bag.
21. Maintain small amount of blood in bottom of prime bag.

    a. Note: discard line should look serosanguinous or darker; if not, you may need to add PRBCs.
    b. Note: two methods can be utilized to add PRBCs.

    - Unspike blood bag from prime filter and elevate filter to let blood drain into prime bag. When complete, clamp tubing as close to bottom of prime bag as possible, then respike the PRBCs bag to keep the spike clean.
    - Add PRBCs into bladder.

22. Circulate until discard line is serosanguinous.
23. Turn off pump.
24. If blood left in prime bag, draw blood out of bladder with 60 mL syringe and save in case additional volume is needed.

    a. Note: open air port on top of prime bag to vent for drainage of bag.
    b. Allow blood to move down venous line to first blue tape (just above ¼, ¼ connector); clamp venous tubing above bridge (at second blue tape below ¼, ¼ connector).

25. Move bridge clamp to arterial tubing and clamp above bridge (at red tape).
26. Hang bridge over pump IV holder (tubing support).
27. Don proper personal protection equipment (PPE), including surgical hat, mask, and gloves when assembling sterile equipment and tubing pack.
28. Disconnect prime lines including ¼, ¼ connectors from patient lines; discard prime setup, keeping sterile.
29. Connect (heavy plastic side on bottom; 3M stamped on this end) CDI cassette to venous line.
30. Connect AV loop venous side (no ¼, ¼ connector) to CDI cassette (no ¼, ¼ connector).

31. Ask ECMO specialist to use 60 mL syringe to push blood prime back from the bladder into the AV loop and prime the SvO_2 sensor.
    a. Note: you need to regulate blood flow by controlling clamp on venous tubing.
32. For airless connection on arterial side, ask specialist to use "needleless" 60 mL syringe of blood and drop blood into tubing on arterial side. Once filled, connect arterial AV loop to arterial tubing on circuit.
33. Remove venous clamp and place on bridge and remove arterial clamp.
34. Turn pump on.
35. Allow flow through newly attached AV loop.
36. Circulate pump slowly (start at 25 mL/min) to see if prime flows through circuit freely.

    a. If prime moves freely, increase flow to 200 mL/k/min (ensures pump and circuit can handle full flow and help debubble circuit). You may have to add blood to bladder to maintain full flow.

37. Once AV loop is connected, check pump controller box:

    a. Silence switches on either side of box should be down/off position.
    b. Silence lights off.
    c. Circuit control in center of box should be in up or midposition, not on override/down position.

38. Test alarms by briefly clamping venous line and listening for circuit alarms.
39. Check green gas line from gas blender is attached to gas inlet of oxygenator.
40. Turn sweep on to 0.2 LPM gas flow with oxygen set 21% FiO_2.
41. Increase sweep at less than the maximum gas flow as rated on oxygenator.

    a. Medtronic 800 oxygenator max sweep = 2.4 LPM place on 2.2 LPM.
    b. Circulate with sweep on for at least five minutes or until blood turns bright red.

42. Turn off sweep.

a. Note: Use of sweep without patient connection may increase O_2 and decrease CO_2 to unsafe levels.

43. Once sweep is off, slow flow to approximately 100 mL/min.
44. Turn oxygen on blender to 100 percent FiO_2.
45. Ensure sweep is off; no oxygen should be going into circuit at this point.
46. Unclamp bridge and clamp arterial and venous lines (specialist may continue low flow through bridge for at least five minutes or until ready for patient connection).
47. Check that bladder is slightly "dimpled" and pulsating.

    a. If bladder not pulsating, place 3 mL of air into outer bladder chamber.
    b. It may be necessary to remove 3 mL of blood from circuit simultaneously.

48. Perform CG8⁺, H/H (full electrolyte panel with pH and ICa^{++}.

    a. Correct low H/H, pH, base deficit >—5 and ICa^{++}.

49. Ensure heater is ON and set to 37°C.
50. Complete safety checklist for all devices.

Device Safety Checklist:

1. CIRCUIT/OXYGENATOR/CANNULA

    (a) Correct tubing pack for weight and flow requirements.
    (b) Tubing pack package integrity without defect and nonexpired.
    (c) All components present in tubing pack without defect (prime bag, CDI cuvette, better bladder, AV loop etc.).
    (d) Oxygenator package integrity without defect and nonexpired.
    (e) Correct-sized cannulas for patient weight and flow requirements.

2. ECMO PUMP CONSOLE

    (a) All components present on pump and are operational.
    (i) CDI, blender, air bubble detector, transonic flowmeter/probe, oxygenator holder, bladder holder, transducer holder, auto syringe (heparin).

(b) Green gas line with filter is connected to blender.
(c) CDI monitor screen illuminates when turned on and passes self-test.
(d) Cincinnati subzero heater cooler is clean and operational. Distilled water is added below mesh grid.
(e) ECMO pump operational when main power buttons depressed. Battery is fully charged.
(f) Speed control knob displays O when turned all the way down; pump operates when increased.
(g) Flow is set to LPM.
(h) ECMO pump cord is labeled and plugged into red emergency power outlet.

2. PRESSURE MONITOR ALARM LIMITS

(a) Bladder pressure low alarm limit is set at—40mm/hg.
(i) High limit is set at _____.
(b) Pre-oxygenator low limit is set at _____.
(i) High limit is set at _____.
(c) Postoxygenator low limit is set at _____.
(i) High limit is set at _____.
(d) Transducers are zeroed and at the level of the bladder and oxygenator.
(e) Occlude venous line above bladder for several seconds to check low bladder pressure alarm. Pump should shut off when negative pressure reaches—40mmHg.

4. AIR BUBBLE DETECTOR

(a) Air bubble detector with correct-sized inserts for patient (1/4 or 3/8).
(b) Alarm test performed with "dummy" tubing.
(c) Alarms activate audibly and illuminates when air is detected.
(d) Alarm silences when Silence depressed.
(e) Alarm resets when Reset depressed.
(f) Jelly applied, detector placed on venous line above the bladder.

5. CIRCUIT SETUP/PRIMING

(a) Perfusionist on call is present.
(b) All connections to pigtails and stopcocks are tight.

(c) Nonmanufactured connections are tie banded.
(d) Circuit is gas primed and crystalloid primed according to protocol.
(e) Blood consent and ECMO consent are signed.
(f) Blood products ordered according to ECMO protocol.
(g) Washed blood order is validated by attending physician.
(h) Circuit is blood primed upon attending physician's orders.
(i) Medications are added to circuit according to protocol.
(j) Perform CG8+, H/H (full electrolyte panel with pH and ICa^{++}).
(k) Correct low H/H, pH, base deficit >—5, and ICa^{++}.
(l) Pump is operational in arterial mode prior to initiating bypass.
(m) Apply jelly and connect transonic flow probe to arterial line above bridge.

Going on ECMO

1. Before cannulating, surgeon will give an order for nurse or ECMO specialist to give heparin to the patient (50-100 units/kg).
2. When the surgeon is ready to connect the circuit to the cannulas,
3. Unclamp the bridge and turn the pump flow down to 50mL/min.
4. Clamp the arterial and venous lines above the bridge.
5. Remove/unpeel the sterile sleeve from the AV loop.
6. Have AV loop ready for surgeon/OR scrub tech.
a. Ask OR tech to support tubing and peel sleeve back toward venous line, maintaining sterility of AV loop.
7. Hand off sterile tubing to the OR scrub tech in a sterile fashion.
8. OR tech will then divide the lines.
9. When surgeon gives order to go on bypass, **turn off pump** and then clamp bridge.
10. Ensure arterial and venous lines are clamped.
11. ECMO primer will remove venous clamp upon surgeon's request to initiate bypass followed by unclamping arterial line; bridge is clamped.
12. When cannulas are connected to AV lines, surgeon will request to initiate bypass.
13. Turn on sweep at 0.5 L/min for Medtronic 800.
14. Start sweep at 1 L/min for Medtronic 1500.
15. Ensure FiO_2 at 70%.
16. Wean FiO_2 and sweep after first blood gas.
17. Begin pump flow slowly at 25 mL/min.

18. Judiciously increase pump flow while closely monitoring patient hemodynamic and electrocardiographic status.
19. Increase flow slowly to 100 mL/kg to ensure nonresistant flow through circuit and cannula.
20. Secure arterial and venous catheters to patient's bed.
21. Maintain flow at 100 mL/kg for five minutes, and if patient is stable

    a. Flash circuit bridge
    b. Check bladder for pulsation
    c. Perform arterial and venous blood gas
    d. Calibrate SVO_2 monitor
    e. Perform $CG8^+$, H/H, and full electrolyte panel with pH and ICa^{++}
    i. Correct low H/H, pH, base deficit >—5, and ICa^{++}
    f. Check platelet count
    g. Correct platelets if < 100,000

Note: Once on, bypass catecholamine washout will occur (the smaller the child, the more severe the reaction), so you may see blood pressure decrease; it should reset itself within a minute or so. If not, give volume.

Circuit Setup: Quadrox Oxygenator / Jostra HL—20 Centrifugal Pump / Better Bladder Box / Transonic Flow Probe

1. Gather equipment—pump with stand, heat exchanger, blender, clamps, tubing pack, appropriate-sized oxygenator, infusion pumps, CDI monitor, Transonic flowmeter, and probe.
2. Check package integrity of ECMO tubing pack and oxygenator for physical defects such as cracked ports, damaged wrap, and patent O_2 ports.
3. Check that pump and electronics are working.
4. Hang Plasmalyte on pump IV pole.
5. Don proper personal protection equipment (PPE), including surgical hat, mask, and gloves when assembling sterile equipment and tubing pack.
6. Have someone open the Quadrox oxygenator box and place in the bracket with the blood outlet on the top (red capped). The writing on outside of oxygenator should be right-side up. Place pigtails top and bottom of oxygenator; make sure stopcocks closed.
7. Have someone open sterile pack and place outer sterile wrap on the floor under the bladder box (to keep tubing that drapes on the floor

sterile). Tighten all pigtails and stopcocks in the tray before removing any tubing.
8. Remove reservoir bag from tray. Hang bag from IV pole using a tubing clamp to hold yellow port top of bag. Clamp discard line and priming solution line (orange filter).
9. Connect venous tubing from bag (blue tape) to venous side of patient bypass bridge (blue tape). Connect arterial tubing from bag (red tape) to arterial side of patient bypass bridge (red tape).
10. Connect venous tubing coming down from patient bridge and ensure no twisting of tubing.
11. Following the lay of the tubing, place pump head cone in pump casing.
12. Blood path must be unobstructed for CO_2 flush and vacuum prime.
13. Connect tubing from pump head cone outlet to oxygenator inlet port at bottom of oxygenator.
14. Heat exchanger water testing. Check for water cleanliness.
15. Fill with distilled or sterile water to fill line (above mesh).
16. Connect water lines to heat exchanger with water going in bottom and coming out top. Direction of water flow must be countercurrent to blood flow for optimal heat exchange. Open the valves and turn on the heater. Never restrict water outlet because it may overpressurize water path and cause water leak. Set heater temperature at 37.5°C. Test heat exchanger for water leaks for at least five minutes.
17. A dry sterile intact circuit may be usable for up to thirty (30) days.

CO_2 Prime

1. Place sterile green gas filter (in the pack) into the line and attach to 100% CO_2 tank (follow flow direction arrow on filter). CO_2 must be filtered with bacteriological filter since it is entering the blood path.
2. Place tubing clamp between upper and lower pigtails prebladder. Open one stopcock on pigtail proximal to clamp (closet to bridge). Place CO_2 line into stopcock on pigtail distal to clamp (before bladder) and open stopcock.
3. Place tubing clamps on patient bypass bridge and the prebypass filter line. Close the clamps on the prime bag discard line and blood prime line (orange filter).
4. Flowmeter on blender *must be off*.
5. Connect gas line green to oxygenator O_2 *inlet* on top of oxygenator. Connect vacuum line to oxygenator O_2 *outlet* (bottom of oxygenator) and clamp.

6. Slowly turn on CO_2 (0.2-0.5 L/min), watching prime bag for filling and listening for CO_2 release out of stopcock. Gas should be turned on just high enough to completely fill prime bag, and primer should be able to hear gas released through stopcock (max 7 L/min). Open clamps on two bypass lines for fifteen seconds to flush out air. CO_2 flush for at least five minutes. (CO_2 flush replaces air with CO_2, making debubbling easier during circuit priming. CO_2 provides a safety mechanism as it is more soluble in blood, so it would be less detrimental to patient in the event that a bubble remained in circuit.)
7. Entire circuit must be closed (except one exit port on prebladder pigtail) for CO_2 to flush air through circuit. After five minutes, turn off CO_2, close CO_2 and release stopcock.
8. Remove clamp from vacuum line (oxygenator outlet) and turn vacuum up to 120-150 mm Hg (vacuum source must not exceed—500 mmHg; membrane rupture may occur). Remove all clamps from circuit. Green tubing should be connected between O_2 inlet (top of oxygenator) and flowmeter. FLOWMETER SHOULD BE OFF. System should be totally closed; prime bag and bladder should collapse immediately if there is no leak in system. Leave vacuum on for at least five minutes.
9. Remove all open stopcock caps and replace with closed caps.

Save the package labels with the lot numbers and expiration dates of all items used. Store in the ECMO cart until the end of the case. Write the date and time the circuit was set up and CO_2 flushed.

Crystalloid Priming

1. Turn pump silence on and override on.
2. Clamp off all outlets from prime bag.
3. Clamp the AV bridge on the circuit and clamp the prebypass filter.
4. Spike the Plasmalyte bag and fill prime bag through blood filter (orange) line. Debubble and bleed out air through stopcock on the top of prime bag.
5. Place clamp just distal to bladder and clamp patient bypass bridge.
6. Open venous line slowly, "walking" fluid toward bladder. Remove air from bladder via stopcock on top of bladder.
7. Check heat exchanger for water leaks (check for moisture in tubing at blood outlet and water check atmospheric vent).
8. Remove tubing clamp from oxygenator inlet, allowing rapid priming of oxygenator and heat exchanger.

9. Remove clamp on ARTERIAL inlet line on bag with prebypass filter.
10. Turn on pump and recirculate through AV loop.
11. Open bridge clamps to debubble bridges.
12. Open stopcocks to debubble pigtails and stopcocks.
13. GENTLY tap oxygenator to remove air using an open hand. Repeat as necessary.
14. Do not exceed 1 L/min flow during priming as a membrane shift could occur after circuit is debubbled; remove vacuum from O_2 outlet.
15. Tie band all positive connections that are not bonded, including heat exchanger outlet. Before banding, be sure that tubing is on connectors as far as they will go.
16. To debubble bridge, turn off pump, unclamp the bridge, and send air up arterial line. Reclamp bridge.
17. Purge all pigtails. Note: When purging pigtails prebladder, the pump must be turned off to avoid negative pressure and air entering venous line.
18. Set up pressure monitors: preoxygenator, postoxygenator, bladder pressure.
19. Prime the preoxygenator and postoxygenator transducers with Plasmalyte.
20. Connect preoxygenator and postoxygenator transducers with an airless connection to the pigtails.
21. Connect the nonfluid-filled bladder pressure transducer connection to the bladder pressure monitor.
22. Connect pressure transducer cables to the appropriate transducers.
23. Zero each pressure transducer and set the high and low limits.
24. Document the date and time the circuit was crystalloid primed, along with all lot numbers and expiration dates.
25. Turn off the pump and remove all the clamps from the circuit if it is not going to be used immediately.

Crystalloid-primed sterile circuit may remain intact for patient use for seven days.

Blood Prime

Supplies Needed

- Neonatal circuit

    - Packed red blood cells (one [1] unit, washed)
    - Heparin (250 units)
        - 250 units = 1/4 mL of 1,000 u/mL
    - Sodium bicarbonate (8% $NaHCO_3$) (10 mEq)
        - 10 mEq = 10 mL
    - Fresh frozen plasma with filter (50 mL)
    - 25 % albumin (25 mL)
    - Calcium chloride (10% $CaCl_2$) (500 mg)
        - 500 mg = 5 mL of 100 mg/mL

- Pediatric / adult circuit

    - Packed red blood cells (one [1] unit, washed)
    - Heparin (500 units)
        - 500 units = 1/2 mL of 1,000 u/mL
    - Sodium bicarbonate (8% $NaHCO_3$) (20 mEq)
        - 20 mEq = 20 mL
    - Fresh frozen plasma with filter (100 mL)
    - 25 % albumin (25 mL)
    - Calcium chloride (10% $CaCl_2$) (1,000 mg)
        - 1,000 mg = 10 mL of 100 mg/mL

1. Turn off pump.
2. Turn on the heater and circulate with the temperature at 37°C.
3. Clamp two (2) outside tubes on prime bag (arterial and venous); leave middle Plasmalyte prime line open. (Note: clamp as close to bag as possible to save blood.)
4. Lower Plasmalyte bag, unclamp, and let prime bag drain into empty Plasmalyte bag.
5. Attach discard line (under prebypass filter) to patient port of a suction canister; leave tubing clamped (leave vacuum port on canister open to air).
6. Attach a 60-cc syringe to bladder stopcock and remove 50 mL of volume from bladder (to prevent dilution of prime); close stopcock.

7. Remove Plasmalyte bag and attach one (1) unit washed PRBCs with a blood filter; open to prime bag and fill prime bag.
8. Make sure tubing from each side of prime bag remains clamped.
9. Have additional washed PRBC quad packs available on unit.
10. Prime venous side first (route of flow) by removing venous clamp closest to prime bag. (Note: when clamp opened, blood will gush and stop at bladder; this is normal.)
11. Clamp venous tubing just before bladder and remove crystalloid from bladder with 60 mL syringe; close stopcock.
12. Unclamp venous line at bladder and discard line to suction canister.
13. Watch blood bag to prevent bag from emptying; observe waste line and until steady stream of prime enters the canister.
14. When blood reaches top of oxygenator, clamp arterial line.
15. Invert bladder.

16. Add medications to bladder *in this order*

   b. Note: volume will increase backward into prime bag; that's okay.

   - Neonatal circuit

      - Heparin (250 units)
         - 250 units = 1/4 mL of 1,000 u/mL
      - Sodium bicarbonate (10 mEq of 8% $NaHCO_3$)
         - 10 mEq = 10 mL
      - 25% albumin (50 mL)
      - Fresh frozen plasma with filter (50 mL)
      - Calcium chloride (10% $CaCl_2$) (500 mg)
         - 500 mg = 5 mL of 100 mg/mL

   - Pediatric / adult circuit

      - Heparin (500 units)
         - 500 units = 1/2 mL of 1,000 u/mL
      - Sodium bicarbonate (20 mEq of 8% $NaHCO_3$)
         - 20 mEq = 20 mL
      - 25% albumin (50 mL)
      - Fresh frozen plasma with filter (100 mL)
      - Calcium chloride (10% $CaCl_2$) (1,000 mg)
         - 1,000 mg = 10 mL of 100 mg/mL

17. Turn off bladder stopcock.
18. Clamp arterial line just above the discard line and open discard line.
19. Turn on pump slowly, approximately 25 mL/min, until blood shows in discard line.
20. Watch priming bag.
21. Maintain small amount of blood in bottom of prime bag.
22. Discard line should look serosanguinous or darker; if not, you may need to add PRBCs.

    i. Note: two methods can be utilized to add PRBCs.

    ii. Unspike blood bag from prime filter and elevate filter to let blood drain into prime bag. When complete, clamp tubing as close to bottom of prime bag as possible, then respike the PRBCs bag to keep the spike clean.
    iii. Add PRBCs into bladder.

23. Circulate until discard line is serosanguinous.
24. Turn off pump.
25. If blood left in prime bag, draw blood out of bladder with 60 mL syringe and save in case additional volume is needed.
26. Note: open air port on top of prime bag to vent for drainage of bag.
27. Allow blood to move down venous line to first blue tape (just above ¼, ¼ connector); clamp venous tubing above bridge (at second blue tape, below ¼, ¼ connector).
28. Move bridge clamp to arterial tubing and clamp above bridge (at red tape).
29. Hang bridge over pump IV holder (tubing support).
30. Don proper personal protection equipment (PPE), including surgical hat, mask, and gloves when assembling sterile equipment and tubing pack.
31. Disconnect prime lines including ¼, ¼ connectors from patient lines; discard prime setup, keeping sterile.
32. Connect (heavy plastic side on bottom; 3M stamped on this end) CDI cassette to venous line.
33. Connect AV loop venous side (no ¼, ¼ connector) to CDI cassette (no ¼, ¼ connector).
34. Ask ECMO specialist to use 60 mL syringe to push blood prime back from the bladder into the AV loop and prime the SvO_2 sensor.
35. Note: you need to regulate blood flow by controlling clamp on venous tubing.

36. For airless connection on arterial side, ask specialist to use "needleless" 60 mL syringe of blood and drop blood into tubing on arterial side. Once filled, connect arterial AV loop to arterial tubing on circuit.
37. Remove venous clamp and place on bridge and remove arterial clamp.
38. Turn pump on.
39. Allow flow through newly attached AV loop.
40. Circulate pump slowly (start at 25 mL/min) to see if prime flows through circuit freely.
41. If prime moves freely, increase flow to 200 mL/k/min (ensures pump and circuit can handle full flow and help debubble circuit); you may have to add blood to bladder to maintain full flow.
42. Once AV loop is connected, check pump controller box: silence switches.
43. Circuit control in center of box should be in override.
44. Test alarms by briefly clamping venous line and listening for circuit alarms.
45. Check green gas line from gas blender is attached to gas inlet of oxygenator.
46. Turn sweep on to 0.2 LPM gas flow with oxygen set 21% FiO_2.
47. Increase sweep at less than the maximum gas flow as rated on oxygenator.

    i. Quadrox Mini max sweep = 2 LPM

48. Circulate with sweep on for at least five minutes or until blood turns bright red.
49. Turn off sweep.
50. Note: Use of sweep without patient connection may increase O_2 and decrease CO2 to unsafe levels.
51. Once sweep is off, slow flow to approximately 100 mL/min.
52. Turn oxygen on blender to 100% FiO_2.
53. Ensure sweep is off; no oxygen should be going into circuit at this point.
54. Unclamp bridge and clamp arterial and venous lines (specialist may continue low flow through bridge for at least five minutes or until ready for patient connection).
55. Check that bladder is slightly "dimpled" and pulsating.
56. If bladder not pulsating, place 3 mL of air into outer bladder chamber.

Extracorporeal Life Support Training Manual

57. It may be necessary to remove 3 mL of blood from circuit simultaneously.
58. Perform CG8⁺, H/H (full electrolyte panel with pH and ICa^{++}).
59. Correct low H/H, pH, base deficit >—5, and ICa^{++}.
60. Ensure heater is ON and set to 37°C.
61. Complete safety checklist for all devices.

Device Safety Checklist

1. CIRCUIT/OXYGENATOR/CANNULA

    a. Correct tubing pack for weight and flow requirements.
    b. Tubing pack package integrity without defect and nonexpired.
    c. All components present in tubing pack without defect (prime bag, CDI cuvette, better bladder, AV loop, etc.).
    d. Oxygenator package integrity without defect and nonexpired.
    e. Correct-sized cannulas for patient weight and flow requirements.

2. ECMO PUMP CONSOLE

    a. All components present on pump and are operational.
    b. CDI, blender, air bubble detector, Transonic flowmeter/probe, oxygenator holder, bladder holder, transducer holder, auto syringe (heparin).
    c. Green gas line with filter is connected to blender.
    d. CDI monitor screen illuminates when turned on and passes self-test.
    e. Cincinnati subzero heater cooler is clean and operational.
    f. Distilled water is added below mesh grid.
    g. ECMO pump operational when main power buttons depressed (Target and M illuminated). Battery is fully charged (C light will not be illuminated).
    h. Speed control knob displays O when turned all the way down; pump operates when increased.
    i. Flow is set to LPM.
    j. ECMO pump cord is labeled and plugged into red emergency power outlet.

3. PRESSURE MONITOR ALARM LIMITS

    a. Bladder pressure low alarm limit is set at—40mm/hg.

i. High limit is set at _____.
 b. Pre-oxygenator low limit is set at _____.
   i. High limit is set at _____.
 c. Post-oxygenator low limit is set at _____.
   i. High limit is set at _____.
 d. Transducers are zeroed and at the level of the bladder and oxygenator.
 e. Occlude venous line above bladder for several seconds to check low bladder pressure alarm. Pump should shut off when negative pressure reaches—40mmHg.

4. AIR BUBBLE DETECTOR

 a. Air bubble detector with correct-sized inserts for patient (1/4 or 3/8).
 b. Alarm test performed with "dummy" tubing.
 c. Alarms activates audibly and illuminates when air detected.
 d. Alarm silences when Silence depressed.
 e. Alarm resets when Reset depressed.
 f. Jelly applied, detector placed on venous line above the bladder.

5. CIRCUIT SETUP/PRIMING

 a. Perfusionist on call is present.
 b. All connections to pigtails and stopcocks are tight.
 c. Nonmanufactured connections are tie banded.
 d. Circuit is gas primed and crystalloid primed according to protocol.
 e. Blood consent and ECMO consent are signed.
 f. Blood products ordered according to ECMO protocol.
 g. Washed blood order is validated by attending physician.
 h. Circuit is blood primed upon attending physician's orders.
 i. Medications are added to circuit according to protocol.
 j. Perform CG8$^+$, H/H (full electrolyte panel with pH and ICa^{++}).
 k. Correct low H/H, pH, base deficit >—5, and ICa^{++}.
 l. Pump is operational in arterial mode prior to initiating bypass.
 m. Apply jelly and connect transonic flow probe to arterial line above bridge.

Going on ECMO

1. Before cannulating, surgeon will give an order for nurse or ECMO specialist to give heparin to the patient (50-100 units/kg).
2. Prior to the surgeon connecting the circuit to the cannulas unclamp the bridge and clamp the arterial and venous lines above the bridge.
3. Turn the pump flow down to 50mL/min.
4. Remove/unpeel the sterile sleeve from the AV loop.
5. Have AV loop ready for surgeon/OR scrub tech.
6. Ask OR tech to support tubing and peel sleeve back toward venous line, maintaining sterility of AV loop.
7. Hand off sterile tubing to the OR scrub tech in a sterile fashion.
8. Surgeon/OR tech will then divide the lines.
9. When surgeon gives order to go on bypass, **turn off pump** and then clamp bridge.
10. Ensure arterial and venous lines are clamped.
11. ECMO primer will remove venous clamp upon surgeon's request to initiate bypass followed by unclamping arterial line; bridge is clamped.
12. When cannulas are connected to AV lines, surgeon will request to initiate bypass.
13. Turn on sweep at 0.5 L/min for Quadrox Mini.
14. Start sweep at 1 L/min for pediatric Quadrox.
15. Ensure FiO_2 at 70%.
16. Wean FiO_2 and sweep after first blood gas.
17. Begin pump flow slowly at 25 mL/min.
18. Judiciously increase pump flow while closely monitoring patient hemodynamic and electrocardiographic status.
19. Increase flow slowly to 100 mL/kg to ensure nonresistant flow through circuit and cannula.
20. Secure arterial and venous catheters to patient's bed.
21. Maintain flow at 100 mL/kg for five minutes, and if patient is stable
    a. Flash circuit bridge
    b. Check bladder for pulsation
    c. Perform arterial and venous blood gas
    d. Calibrate SVO_2 monitor
    e. Perform CG8[+], H/H, and full electrolyte panel with pH and ICa^{++}

f. Correct low H/H, pH, base deficit >—5, and ICa^{++}
   g. Check platelet count
      i. Correct if < 100,000

Note: Once on, bypass catecholamine washout will occur (the smaller the child, the more severe the reaction), so you may see blood pressure decrease; it should reset itself within a minute or so. If not, give volume.

Chapter 4

Medical Preparations Precannulation

Heparin Loading Dose

The heparin loading dose is prepared by the pharmacy. Give the heparin loading dose to the patient during the cannulation procedure. Give dose under direct verbal instruction of the cannulating surgeon. As a loading dose, the patient receives 50-100 units per kilogram of heparin. The bolus is given via central line access and flushed with 3 mL of normal saline. The dose must be verified and signed by two licensed staff members.

Documentation

The ECMO specialist must complete the checklist once the priming procedure is complete. A detailed narrative and assessment note must also be written on the flow sheet. All relevant calculations must also be documented on the flow sheet. Vital signs and other entries begin once the cannulation procedure is started. Blood products administered are to be entered onto the blood utilization section of the flow sheet.

Narrative Note

A narrative note is required at the beginning of every shift. Documentation from that point on through the shift is to be under certain circumstances as listed.

a. ECMO Start-Up Note

This note is to be written at the initiation of an ECMO. It should include the following:

1. Perfusionist or ECMO priming specialist present.
2. Time started.
3. Safety check completed.
4. HOSPITAL tubing pack used, expiration, and size (1/4" or 3/8").
5. Oxygenator size, serial number, expiration.
6. SVO_2 monitor calibrated as per protocol.
7. Medications added, specific name and amount.
8. Heparin bolus given, amount.
9. Blood products used and their donor numbers.
10. Pre-ACT, pre-ABG, H/H, platelets, and patient vital signs.
11. Therapeutics given.
12. Heparin drip checked and connected to circuit.
13. Cannulae's sizes and site.
14. Surgeons present and procedure performed under sterile conditions.
15. Time on bypass, how tolerated.
16. Serial number from oxygenator and tubing pack should be documented in the patient's record.

b. Initial Assessment Note

This note should include a minimum amount of information that is patient related, mainly concentrating on pump-related information.

i. Neurological assessment (pupils, fontanel)
ii. Respiratory assessment (breath sounds)
iii. Cannulae site
iv. Other invasive sites that may be hemorrhaging
v. Any lines that may be in the circuit
vi. Circuit assessment (checklist complete, abnormal findings)
vii. Perfusionist or ECMO priming specialist on call
viii. Intensivist/fellow in house on call
ix. Surgical attending/fellow on call

c. Daily Events

These are events that require a narrative note.

1. Blood product transfusion—All blood products given must be documented with their donor numbers (if applicable) and their justification for administration under concurrent blood utilization. The date of expiration should also be included as part of the documentation.
2. Flow Difficulties—All instances of chattering and others must be documented with treatment given.
3. Circuit Procedures—Such as emergencies, stopcock changes, etc., must be documented. Emergency documentation must contain equipment and materials used, perfusionist backup notified, Intensivist notified, and how the emergency was handled.

ECMO ADMISSION ORDERS

1. Admit to PICU and transfer to ECLS (extracorporeal life support) service.
2. Neonatal patients on ECMO warmer bed with infant servo control (ISC) probe.
3. Place neonatal patients on special neonatal mattress.
4. Pediatric patients on ECMO specialty bed with RIK mattress.
5. Neonatology consult for neonates.
6. Pediatric surgical consult.
7. Vital signs (temperature, HR, BP, CVP, RR, SAO2 [pre and post ductal] Q 1 hour.
8. Place head midline and elevated thirty degrees.
9. Record admission weight, height, abdominal girth, and head circumference.
10. Daily abdominal girth.
11. Daily head circumference.
12. Foley catheter to urimeter. Monitor and record Intake and output hourly. Record and evaluate daily cumulative intake and output balance.
13. Hematest all stools and record results.
14. NPO, nasogastric, or oral gastric tube to gravity.

Diagnostics

17. Daily brain ultrasound if less than eight months of age
18. Echocardiogram to evaluate cardiac function during ECMO

19. Daily portable chest x-ray at 0600
20. Chromosomes on admission for congenital diaphragmatic hernia (CDH) patients

Laboratory

21. Blood culture (central line if available) upon admission
22. Urine culture (catheter if available) upon admission
23. Endotracheal culture
24. P8, iCa$^+$, H/H, platelet count on arrival, then q 6 hours for 48 hours, then q 12 hours if stable
25. Mg, PO4, T&D bilirubin on arrival, then q 12 hours for 48 hours, then q day and PRN if stable (bilirubin for newborn patients only
26. Antithrombin III level q 12 h and prn
27. CBC with differential, PT, PTT, heparin level, antifactor Xa, fibrinogen, and fibrin split products daily
28. Colloid oncotic pressure daily
29. Activated clotting time (ACT) q 30 minutes until stable then q 1 hour
30. ABGs with each ventilator change and every 4 hours for 48 hours, then every 8 hours
31. ECMO pump gases (preoxygenator and postoxygenator) every 8 hours and PRN
32. TEG daily in morning
33. RECORD ALL BLOOD DRAWS ML FOR ML and record cumulative daily total

Blood Bank

34. Please order all blood products leukodepleted and CMV safe
35. Only order irradiated blood products if specified by MD and patient has history of bone marrow transplant (BMT), history of Immunosuppression, or diagnosis of DiGeorge syndrome
36. Two (2) units PRBCs (one [1] unit washed, one [1] unit quadpacked if for an infant for cannulation
37. Two (2) units PRBCs on hold for ECMO, one (1) unit quadpacked if for an infant for cannulation at all times
38. One (1) unit FFP for cannulation
39. One (1) unit FFP on hold for ECMO at all times
40. Two (2) units platelets for cannulation
41. Two (2) units platelets on hold for ECMO at all times

Extracorporeal Life Support Training Manual

42. Please notify the *hospital* blood bank when the patient is decannulated so blood products are no longer kept on hold

Intravenous

43. D10W + 5,000 units heparin/50mL - ECMO circuit as per protocol
44. Heparin loading dose (precannulation) _____units (50-100mg/kg)
45. .45 Sodium Chloride + 1 unit heparin/mL at 1mL/hr (arterial line/UAL)
46. .45 sodium chloride + 1 unit heparin /mL at 1mL hr (central venous line/UVL)
47. .2 sodium chloride + 1 meq KCL/100mL_____(80 mL/kg/day < 12 kg)
48. .45 sodium chloride + 2 meq KCL/100mL _____(60 mL/kg/day > 12kg)

Medications

49. Ampicillin IV (200 mg/kg/day) divided q6h_____

50. Gentamicin IV (4 mg/kg/dose)

    i. >34 wks-3months
    ii. Q 24h (newborn 0-7 days) _____
    iii. Q 12h (newborn > 7 days) _____

51. Ceftriaxone IV (100 mg/kg/day)

    i. > 3 months
    ii. Q 12 h _____

52. Fentanyl IV (2 microgram/kg)

    i. Bolus _____

53. Fentanyl IV (1-2 microgram/kg/hr)

    i. Continuous infusion _____

54. Norcuran IV (0.1 mg/kg/hr) _____

i. Titrate to a 2/4 "train of four"

55. Ativan IV (0.1 mg/kg/hr)

i. Continuous infusion _____

ECMO Circuit

56. Calculate therapeutic extracorporeal flow rate _____ mL/min (70-120mL/kg/min)
57. Continuous preoxygenator/postoxygenator pressure monitoring and document q 1 hour
58. Continuous bladder pressure monitoring and document q 1 hour
59. Continuous SVO_2, hemoglobin, and hematocrit monitoring and document q 1 hour
60. Calibrate CDI-100 monitor q 8 hrs with preoxygenator blood gas sample and patient CBC
61. Daily ECMO parameters to be written by ECMO physician
62. Specialist circuit safety Check q 6 hours and record

Initial (PRE-ECMO) Ventilator Settings

63. Conventional

FiO_2: ____ IMV: ____ PIP: ____ PEEP: ____ VT: ____

64. High Frequency

FiO_2: ____ HZ: ____ AMP: ____ PEEP: ____ MAP: ____

RESTING SETTINGS

65. Conventional

FiO_2: ____ IMV: ____ PIP: ____ PEEP: ____ VT: ____

66. High Frequency

FiO_2: ____ HZ: ____ AMP: ____ PEEP: ____ MAP: ____

EMERGENCY VENTILATOR SETTINGS

67. Conventional

FiO_2: ____ IMV: ____ PIP: ____ PEEP: ____ VT: ____

68. High Frequency

FiO_2: ____ HZ: ____ AMP: ____ PEEP: ____ MAP: ____

69. Aerosal Treatments: _____

VITAL SIGNS PARAMETERS
(notify house officer with any changes)

70. HR _____ TO _____
    BP _____ TO _____
    RR _____ TO _____
    MAP _____ TO _____

71. Physical therapy consult for positioning
72. Social work consult (notified date and time)

_____

Chapter 5

Cannulation

During the cannulation procedure, the ECMO specialist, perfusionist, or ECMO priming specialist will continually monitor the pump. Final entries about the priming procedure are done. The pump blood results including pH, H/H, blood gas, and electrolytes are treated if needed. The cannulae and cannulae connectors are given to the surgeon/OR nurse. Once the actual connection of the circuit is started, the perfusionist is responsible for actually coordinating the connection. Vital signs are closely monitored during this phase. Once cannulation is complete, blood flow will be initiated upon orders from the surgeon.

Cannulation Process

It is strongly recommended that the **team** *creates an accurate, complete, and active process of* **all** *activities to improve and maintain quality.*

Cannulation

Document

1. Vital signs every fifteen minutes (HR, B/P, CVP, SaO_2) until cannulation completed, then every thirty minutes.
2. Don proper personal protection equipment (PPE), including surgical hat, mask, and gloves when assembling sterile equipment and tubing pack.
3. Sterile technique observed; surgical attire in use.
4. Secure catheters to bed.

5. Personnel involved with procedure.
6. Use of safety checklists.
7. Time of paralyzation/sedation.
8. Time of heparinization.
9. Ventilator changes.
10. Patient's tolerance to procedure.

Initiating VA Bypass

Once the cannulae are connected and the circuit is checked for air, the perfusionist and/or the ECMO specialist will initiate bypass upon the order of the surgeon. This is done in the following manner:

1. ECMO blood flow is started at 25 mL/minute and increased full flow within two to three minutes depending on the tolerance of the patient until a flow 100 mL/kg/min is reached (maximum calculated flow is 150 mL/kg/min). Flow should be increased to 140 mL/kg/min transiently within the first fifteen to twenty minutes to ensure circuit and cannula stability. Note: in the case of myocardial stun, the flow may need to be increased at a faster rate as the baby is now dependent upon the cardiac support as well as the respiratory support.
2. ACTs are performed immediately and then every fifteen minutes until stable. The heparin drip is started at 0.51 mL/hour once the ACTs drop to < 400 seconds.
3. A complete set of labs should be sent as soon as possible. These include CBC, platelets, P8, ICa, Mg, PO3, PT, PTT, FDP, fibrinogen, blood cultures.
4. During bypass, platelets will be administered *postoxygenator* to the patient if necessary.
5. An in vivo calibration for SvO_2 is performed. This should be done once full flow is reached. The pump gases should be done as soon as possible.
6. Once full flows are reached and the patient is stable, the patient may be placed on resting ventilator settings. The patient is usually weaned to these settings over thirty minutes. An emergency settings card is written and placed on the patient's ventilator.

Suggested Rest Ventilator Settings

Conventional
FiO_2:   21-.30

PIP: 10 cm H$_2$0
PEEP: 10 cm H$_2$0
IMV: 10 BPM
Ti: 3-5 seconds

Suggested High Frequency Ventilator Settings

FiO$_2$: .21-.30
Hz: 15
AMP: 25

7. Prebypass vasopressors may now be weaned and discontinued per physician's orders. The physician may elect to leave a low dose of cardiotropic medication (dopamine infusing 3-5 mcg/kg/min).
8. An echocardiogram for specific placement of the ECMO cannulae's may be required.

Initiating VV-ECMO Bypass

Initial catheter placement and function is crucial in VV-ECMO for venous return and arterial flow. The biomedicus arterial return catheter portion must be placed cephalic (up over the head), behind and against the ear, and secured. This places the arterial port facing the tricuspid valve. The tip of the end of the catheter should remain approximately 1 cm above the diaphragm. Head, neck, and shoulder position affect the catheter function. Intrathoracic pressure changes affect catheter tip position and function. Right atrial volume and cardiac output affect catheter function, venous return, and recirculation.

Begin flows at 10 mL/kg/min and increase slowly to 100-140 mL/kg/min. Saturation of venous and arterial blood may decrease as right atrial volume decreases or due to poor catheter position. Intracardiac filling (preload) and cardiac function must be maintained. Increasing VV flows may initially increase pulmonary blood flow and create pulmonary congestion/edema, pulmonary hypertension, or decreasing arterial and venous saturation.

Primary Nurse Responsibility

The primary nurse is responsible for setting up the appropriate bed spot. Warmers and specialty beds and mattresses should be used whenever available.

Specific items needed for the ECMO patients are the following:

1. IV neuromuscular agent and sedative boluses for anesthesia
2. IV neuromuscular agent and sedative infusions
3. Analgesia

    a. Fentanyl 2-5 mcg/kg bolus IV PRN during cannulation

        i. Fentanyl will be absorbed by membrane oxygenators and circuits.
        ii. Fentanyl requires initial and repeated bolusing for therapeutic effect.

    b. Norcuran 0.1 mg/kg bolus IV PRN during cannulation
    c. Ativan 0.1 mg/kg bolus IV PRN for cannulation

4. Crystalloid and blood volume boluses

    a. Primary nurse is responsible for maintaining large bore extension tubing with syringes for IV bolus resuscitation.
    b. Primary nurse is responsible for acquiring PRBCs, FFP, albumin, and crystalloid bolus-infusion syringes during the procedure.

Patient Management

Goals

1. ACTs between 160 and 180 utilizing the I-Stat System

    a. ACT management is circuit and flow dependent

        i. Larger more complicated circuits need higher flows
        ii. Oxygenators may be rated for minimum flow
        iii. Circuits may contain coatings that alter coagulation

2. AV-ECMO

    a. paO_2 = 60-80 mmHg
    b. pH = 7.35-7.45
    c. pCO_2 = 35-45
    d. HgB = 13-15

e. Hct > 40
   f. Platelet > 100,000

3. VV-ECMO

   a. paO_2 = 45-80 mmHg
   b. pH = 7.35-7.45
   c. pCO_2 = 35-45
   d. Hgb = 15
   e. Hct > 45
   f. Platelet > 100,000

4. Urine output = > 2 mL/kg/hr
5. Follow daily care plan
6. Heparin drip minimum 25 u/kg
7. Reducing heparin requires approval of medical director

AV-ECMO Flow

1. Flow = 10 mL/kg/min.
2. Regulate ECMO flow to maintain venous saturation of 70%-75%.
3. Flows should not fall below 100 mL/min on a Medtronic 0800 oxygenator.
4. Flows should not fall below 500 mL/min utilizing Jostra HL—20 centrifugal pump and Quadrox oxygenator.

Open Bridge ECMO flows to the patient can be maintained at lower flows than rated flows for the oxygenator or pump by partially occluding the bridge with a clamp to allow exact regulated recirculation through the bridge.

5. This will maintain higher intracircuit flows and deliver specific patient flows.
6. In general, the flow should not be increased or decreased rapidly when changes are made. Flow changes should be in increments of 10-20 mL/min.
7. Regulate sweep gas to maintain ordered parameters for $PaCO_2$.
8. Regulate sweep gas oxygen concentration to maintain patient paO_2 < 100 mmHg (torr).
9. Medtronic oxygenator pressure gradient should not exceed 300 mmHg.

VV-ECMO Flow

1. Flow = 100-140 mL/kg/min.
2. Regulate flow to maintain true mixed venous saturation 65%-85%.
3. Monitor difference between arterial and venous circuit saturations.
4. Calculate "recirculation fraction."
5. Calculate "effective flow."
6. Manage pulse-oximeter saturation and true arterial blood gas measurements.
7. Monitor cephalic saturations.
8. Monitor catheter position.
9. Monitor right arterial filling and cardiac output.
10. Monitor serum-free hemoglobin.

Fluid and Electrolytes

1. Fluid maintenance = 80-120 mL/kg/day
2. 60-80 calories/kg/day
3. Na 2-4 meq/kg/day
4. K 2-3 meq/kg/day
5. Estimated fluid loss from membrane is 50 mL/day. This should be taken into consideration when totaling intake and output.
6. Monitor calcium and magnesium during the use of diuretics.
7. Maintain > 2 cc/kg/hr of urine output with hemofilter or diuretics.
8. Monitor daily total fluid balance to avoid relevant fluid accumulation and edema.

Rapid infusion of any substance, colloid or pharmacological, will alter the oxygenation of the ECLS patient. The ECLS circuit has a fixed volume. **Any** acute change in volume can alter the oxygen delivery due to a change in pulmonary blood flow. By infusing platelets in 10 mL increments followed by a bolus of heparin, the SvO2 may drop, and the patient will require an increase in extracorporeal flow rate. Continuous slow infusion of platelets, with a compensatory increase in heparin, will smoothly change the platelet level and not alter the oxygen consumption and delivery.

Fluid output includes blood, urine, tube drainage, skin loss, pulmonary loss, and oxygenator evaporation. Loss through the Medtronic lung is about 2 mL water/M^2/hr. Fluid intake should balance output. It includes blood products, flush solution, medications, IV fluids, and the heparin drip.

Electrolytes should be maintained at normal levels. Potassium loss and sodium retention frequently occur. Average replacements for full-term infants on ECMO would be the following:

Na	2-4 mEq/kg/day
K+	2-3 mEq/kg/day
Ca++	30-50 mg/kg/day
Mg++	20 mEg/kg/day

In addition, glucose must be supplied as $D_{10}W$ to $D_{15}W$ (80-100 mL/kg/day). Serum electrolytes, Ca levels (as ionized calcium), and glucose levels should be monitored every twelve hours. Bedside Dextrostix can also be done. If the serum-glucose level is elevated, switching the maintenance, heparin, and flush solutions to a lesser concentration of dextrose may be recommended.

Hyperalimentation is usually begun on the second day of ECMO. It should be a nonheparinized solution.

Decreased pulsatile pressure during pass may lead to a decreased glomerular filtration rate and increased renin production. Decreased urinary output is common for morbidly ill patients and patients on bypass.

Lasix (.1-.2 mg/kg/hr IV) is often needed in the following circumstances:

- Decreased urine output (less than 1 mL/kg/hr)
- Elevated blood pressure
- Increased positive fluid balance
- Excessive weight gain

Drug Therapy

1. Heparin drip at 25-60 units/kg/hour. If change is > 10 u/kg, MD will be notified (see heparin management and coagulation performance improvement tool).
2. Prophylactic antibiotics.
3. Anticonvulsants as needed.
4. Narcotics as needed. (Fentanyl 2-5 mcg/kg/min IV, membrane oxygenator, and circuit absorbs Fentanyl. This will prevent achieving therapeutic levels until membrane is saturated. This may require an initial additional 3-10 mcg/kg. The membrane saturation requires individual titration. Attention to blood pressure and myocardial dysfunction.)

5. Sedative/anticonvulsant as needed (Ativan 0.1 mg/kg/hr IV has less cardiovascular side effects).
6. Paralytic agents as needed.

Daily Management

1. ACTs q30 minutes unless stable then q 1 hour
2. ABGs q4 hours until stable then q 8h
3. SVO_2 monitor: continuous, maintain 70%-75%
4. Patient temperature 36.5°C-37°C
5. Daily CXR and brain ultrasounds

O_2/CO_2 Management

The gas delivered to the membrane oxygenator can be controlled and adjusted by several parameters. This will directly manage the patient oxygen and carbon dioxide.

1. FiO_2—The Fraction of Inspired Oxygen is the oxygen composition of the gas being delivered to the **oxygenator and ventilator**. This is expressed as the Fraction of Inspired Oxygen.

   i. FiO_2 should be **increased in the face of hypoxia** PaO_2 < 60 mmHg, MVO_2 < 65 % when the maximum ECMO flow has been achieved.
   ii. FiO_2 should be **decreased when the patient shows hyperoxia** PaO_2 > 100 and when the minimum acceptable extracorporeal flow rate has been attained.

   MVO_2 should be maintained between > 60 and < 80.

2. Gas Flow ("Sweep")
   The delivery rate of flow of the gas through the blender is measured by liters per minute or tenths of a liter. Special blenders for ECLS incorporate .1-liter adjustments.

   - The rate of flow of gas will correlate directly with the gas carbon dioxide to blood carbon dioxide difference.
   - Increasing sweep increases the gas-to-blood difference and reduces the amount of carbon dioxide in the blood.

- Decreasing sweep decreases the gas-to-blood difference and does not reduce the cause the amount of carbon dioxide to be as reduced.
- Sweep is used to flush CO_2 from the circuit and should never be adjusted below zero.
- The gas is blended with the FiO_2 line, which normalizes the $PaCO_2$.
- The respirator should be at minimal support, and the minimum acceptable extracorporeal flow rate has been attained, and the $PaCO_2$ is < ordered by MD. Adjustment of gas sweep with 100% FiO_2 should normalize both paO_2 and $paCO_2$ in the patient with respiratory failure.
- Questions that should be addressed when considering adjustments of the sweep gas are the following:
    - Is the sweep at the minimum or maximum percentage allowed for the oxygenator being used? (See package inserts for specific manufacturers recommendations.)
        - Medtronic 0800 ECMO lung can be adjusted to .5 LPM minimum.
        - All other larger Medtronic oxygenator will use a minimum sweep of 1 LPM.
    - Is the extracorporeal flow rate maintaining a normal SvO_2?
        - If SvO_2 is above parameters, wean the blood flow rate to normalize the SvO_2. A decrease in ECFR will have an effect on the total carbon dioxide volume available for extracorporeal removal.
    - Is the patient on ECLS for cardiac support?
        - If so, the patient may have normal lungs and normal gas exchange. Twenty-one percent oxygenation is often used in this situation, but overventilation may inadvertently take place with normal lungs.
    - Is the patient's ventilator on rest settings?
    - Can the ventilation be lowered without compromising the inflation of the patient's lungs?

- o Is the flowmeter accurate?
- o Is the membrane receiving the appropriate rated flow of blood?

  - **Rated flow** is the flow rate at which venous blood beginning with a saturation of 75% will be fully saturated to 95% at the outlet of the membrane lung.

- o Is the amount of oxygen delivered per minute when running at rated flow?

  - **Maximal O_2 membrane delivery is the amount of oxygen delivered per minute when the oxygenator is being perfused at the rated flow.**

- o Is the membrane efficiency or CO_2 clearance decreased?

  - The change in temperature across the membrane between the warm blood and cool gas may cause condensation to accumulate on the gas side of the membrane surface.
  - The sweep gas flow rate is usually sufficient to maintain the functional surface, but condensation may affect the gas exchange properties of primarily a silicone or nonporous membrane.
  - A technique known as **burbing** the membrane may increase the efficiency of gas exchange.

    - This must be done carefully to avoid an extreme increase in internal membrane pressures that may cause gas emboli into the blood path! This is only a recommendation and should only be performed by someone with extensive experience! Consult medical director or perfusionist before burbing a porous membrane!
    - A cleaned gloved finger is placed firmly over the gas outlet port on the bottom of the membrane with the sweep on two (2) l/m for three (3) seconds to completely restrict the escape of gas flow. When released, this should result in a sudden release of gas and decrease the internal humidity, decrease the

water barrier that may have developed, and improve the membrane blood-gas exchange.
- This condensation generally does not affect the CO_2.

Patient Blood Gases

VA-ECMO

- The patient pO_2 is determined by the ECMO blood flow rates.
  - One should remember the house rule: *"If the O's is low, turn up the flow" (on VA ECMO)*. In doing this, you have allowed more of the cardiac output to be taken over by the ECMO pump, and thus, more of the blood will be fully oxygenated.
  - The patient cardiac output perfuses the lungs, which, when diseased, will not adequately contribute to oxygenation and will most likely result in the desaturation of the blood.
- The membrane, when run at the rated flow and sweep, has maximally saturated the blood, so increasing the gas flow or the FiO_2 to the membrane will not increase the patient's oxygenation.
- The membrane surface area can be a factor in oxygenation or ventilation if a clinically relevant area is lost due to clotting or water vapor formation.
- If the patient's total O_2 consumption exceeds the rated flow of the membrane, you will not oxygenate the patient. Therefore, an appropriate-size membrane must be applied to the expected O_2 consumption.
- If the patient's total CO_2 production exceeds the sweep flow of the membrane, you may need to apply more ventilatory support to the patient. Therefore, an appropriate-size membrane must be applied to the expected CO_2 production.

VV-ECMO

- The oxygenation on VV-ECMO is more dependent on the native lung function. Oxygen delivery to the right atrium is limited to membrane size and amount of gas exchange with pump flow.
- Increasing pump flow more than 140 cc/kg/min usually results in increased recirculation. Recirculation of venous blood in the ECMO

circuit does not improve arterial oxygenation. Recirculation may lower venous CO_2 and arterial CO_2.
- Careful management of native lung function is necessary. Increasing sweep will decrease CO_2 returning to the lungs.
- Arterial content of oxygen and carbon dioxide will be more dependent on intrapulmonary mixing.

Daily Parameters

The daily parameters set by the ECMO physician will determine the patient's blood gas expectations.

paO_2

- The first one to two days, the paO_2 is usually maintained between 80 and 90 torr.
- The MVO_2 is set at 66%-80%.
- Clinical improvement will be expressed by an increase in the MVO_2 or the paO_2 or both.
- If the goal is set at 80-90 torr, then a paO_2 of 100 would direct a decrease of 10-20 mL of ECMO pump blood flow.
- This should continue until the ECMO pump flow rate is at "idle."
- Improving patient paO_2s may mean that the patient's lung gas exchange is improving and/or that pulmonary hypertension is decreasing.
- An increase in MVO_2 (with constant DO_2) is a measurement of decreased oxygen extraction.

    o This may signal an improvement in the metabolic condition of the patient.
        - Weaning the ECMO pump flow is indicated if MVO_2 > 80%.
    o This may be evidence of excessive DO_2.
        - Weaning the ECMO pump flow is indicated if MVO_2 > 80%.
    o This may be evidence of a failure of utilization.
        - Distributive shock (sepsis) / metabolic derangement.
        - Determine etiology of increased MVO_2.
            - Acidosis, decreased urine output, shock may be present.
        - Weaning the ECMO pump flow is not indicated.

paCO$_2$

- Patient paCO$_2$ is primarily maintained by the ECMO membrane gas flow.
    - To decrease paCO$_2$ levels
        - Increase total gas flow
        - Decrease the concentration of CO$_2$ gas going into the membrane
- The infant's respiratory center in the brain will "see" the "pump" paCO$_2$ directly on AV-ECMO because the pump blood is returned into the aortic arch, location of the carotid body, and it will respond to this level and not to the patient paCO$_2$.

    - Therefore, if the pump paCO$_2$ is less than 35 torr, the infant's internal drive to breath is turned off.

- Low ECMO blood flow may also increase patient paCO$_2$s. The treatment is to increase the pump CO$_2$ to stimulate the patient to breathe.
- Low ECMO blood flows (i.e., less than 50% cardiac output), the patient should be breathing or supported by the ventilator.
- If you are only on 50% bypass and the blood gas deteriorates
    - Increase the ECMO flow if patient is fully ventilated and not breathing
        - This is an extremely important concept. It is the tendency to decrease the paCO$_2$ in the pump gas when a high CO$_2$ is seen, and if the high CO$_2$ is the result of decreased respirations, lowering the pump paCO$_2$ will only worsen the process.
- **Note:** A pump gas must be obtained if an unusual patient gas is obtained to assure effective therapy.

Heparin Management

- Systemic (unfractionated) heparin is continuously provided in whatever dose is required to maintain the whole blood activated clotting time (ACT) at 160-180 seconds (I Stat) or approximately 1½ times normal.
- This generally requires 25-60 units/kg/hr of heparin.
    - More or less, dosing is evidence coagulation imbalance.
- Heparin is bound.
    - To platelets and protein.

- o Excreted in the urine, excretion is increased with diuretics and the hemofilter.
- Higher heparin dosages are required during platelet transfusions and diuresis
  - o Lasix increases the excretion of heparin.

- Lower heparin doses may be required during oliguria and anuric renal failure.
- In determining efficiency of anticoagulation, the heparin effect rather than the exact heparin level is the clinical parameter followed.
- Heparin efficiency is measured in whole blood (whole blood activated clotting time [ACT]) rather than plasma (such as partial thromboplastin time or thrombin time). This is not an exact test of heparin but a patient trend that is measured to monitor the clinical condition during bypass. The measurement is less exactly quantitative but critically important to trend. Large persistent changes and measurements should be clinically responded to.
- Direct measurements of heparin levels—antithrombin III (ATIII), PT/PTT, thromboelastograms (TEG)—and evidence of clinical bleeding or clotting should be monitored.
- Heparin requires ATIII to be clinical effective, and low serum levels of ATIII, typically found in sick newborns, will reduce the heparin function and cause **decreasing** ACT measurements in the face of **increasing** heparin dosing.

  - o **Decreasing ACT measurement with increasing heparin doses signals low ATIII levels!**

- ATIII is bound by the newer membrane and circuit coating and may require continuous monitoring and replacement.

Membrane Oxygenator Monitoring

Pressure / Resistance

- Poiseuille's law
- Pressure = flow × resistance
- Pressure drop—the difference between the inlet and outlet pressures
- Delta P = P1—P2 compares to baseline
- Delta P should normally be 0-200 mmHg (Medtronic)
- Delta P should not exceed 300 mmHg (Medtronic)

- Inlet pressure should not exceed 700 mmHg (Medtronic)
- Outlet pressure should not exceed 400 mmHg (Medtronic)
- Transmembrane pressure = pressure gas phase + pressure blood phase
- Transmembrane pressure normally 400 mmHg (Medtronic)
- Transmembrane pressure should not exceed 750 mmHg (Medtronic)
- Increases in membrane pressures may be caused by
  - A clamped line
  - Exceeding rated flow
  - Clots

Flow / Compliance
C= delta Q/ delta P
C= compliance
Q = flow
P = pressure

If compliance of membrane is constant, changes in flow will cause fluctuations in pressure in the oxygenator.

If compliance of membrane is constant, changes in pressure will cause fluctuations in flow in the oxygenator.

If compliance of membrane changes this will cause fluctuations in pressure or flow through the oxygenator.

If flow is constant, changes in pressure will cause fluctuations in compliance in the oxygenator.

If pressure is constant, changes in flow will cause fluctuations in compliance in the oxygenator.

Oxygenation

- Blood flows are laminar and countercurrent to the gas flow.
- Gas diffuses across the membrane due to pressure gradients between the gas flowing and the blood flowing through the membrane (Henry's law of gas diffusion).
- Effectors of the rate of O_2 and CO_2 transfer membrane permeability; silicone is six times more permeable to CO_2 than O_2 and eleven times more permeable to CO_2 than N_2.
- Gas diffusion rate in blood; CO_2 is twenty times more diffusible than O_2.
  - Factors

    c. Membrane surface area
    d. Blood path transient time
    e. Gas path transient time
    f. Partial pressure gradient

Membrane Oxygen Transfer

Membrane (AV) O_2 transfer = $(SAO_2 - SVO_2)(1.34 \times Hgb) \times \text{flow}/100$

Medtronic 800 O_2 transfer = 60-70 mL O_2/M_2/min

Gas Membrane Pressure Monitoring

- All membrane oxygenators have a rated pressure drop across the oxygenating compartment. If this pressure is exceeded, the membrane will fail and rupture during the ECMO procedure.
- The degree of pressure drop is indicative of the amount of resistance to blood flow produced by the oxygenator. It is determined by subtracting the outlet pressure from the inlet pressure. For example, if the inlet pressure is 100 mmHg and the outlet pressure is 60 mmHg, then the pressure drop across the membrane would be 40 mmHg.
- The blood inlet pressure should always be greater than the blood outlet pressure with a gradient of approximately 50-150 mmHg at any one time. Changes of the inlet-outlet pressure gradient during the ECMO procedure may be an early indication of a failing oxygenator.
- NOTE: Clots in the oxygenator result only in a rise of the premembrane pressure.
- The pressure drops or levels of resistance in the ECMO circuit are also cumulative. They may be produced by various physical limitations such as length and size of tubing used, cannulae, or gas pressure. The pressure drop is also affected by blood flow rate, viscosity, and temperature. The postmembrane pressure reflects the sum of these pressures.
- The resistance of the arterial catheter and problems with the arterial line such as kinking, clots, or sutures tied too tight are reflected in a rise of both the postmembrane pressure and premembrane pressure. Postmembrane pressures over 300 mmHg may cause hemolysis or may cause leaking around the tie bands. Pressure greater than 500 mmHg can cause the circuit to explode.
- **Note:** Causes for unusually high postmembrane pressures are the following:

1. Kinked arterial line or catheter
2. Clotted arterial line or catheter
3. Catheter tied too tight
4. Flow too high for the size of arterial catheter
5. Catheter against wall of aorta or dissection of aortic arch
6. Clotted heat exchanger

- Premembrane and postmembrane pressures must be measured and charted every eight hours. Any sudden change or steady increase in pressure must be reported to the ECMO physician and perfusionist on call. **Accurate adjustment of the high-pressure alarm on the pressure monitor will alert the specialist to problems as it happens.**
- The pressure gradient across the membrane should be less than the following:

  - 150 mmHg for the 0800 or 1,500 membranes
  - 250 mmHg for the Ultrox membranes
  - If the postmembrane pressure rises above 300 mmHg, the ECMO physician and perfusionist on call must be notified.

Tie Banding

All connections on the arterial side of the pump should be tie banded when setting up the circuit. A tie band should also be placed on all connections not made by the manufacturer. A tie band should be placed on the outlet to the bladder when the connection from the tubing to the bladder is made.

Care of a Patient on ECMO

The care of the patient on ECMO is essentially the same as the care of any critically ill patient who requires intensive medical and nursing management. The added care involved is the ECMO circuit, primarily the responsibility of the ECMO specialist.

Documentation

ECMO Specialist

General Statements

1. ECMO utilizes twenty-four-hour flow sheets. All totals are zeroed at 0730.
2. Military time is to be used.
3. All charting is to be done in permanent ink.
4. All flow sheets are to be signed.
5. Dates are to appear on all flow sheets.
6. All flow sheets are to be stamped with the patient nameplate.
7. All procedures performed on the ECMO circuit are to be charted here.

    i. *Code* refers to code descriptions to be charted when performed.
    ii. ECMO

    a. Temp. pt.—refers to patient temperature
    b. Temp. H_2O—refers to temperature of water heater
    c. Flow—refers to the rate at which blood flows through the pump tubing, regulated by pump
       A = actual C = calculated flow
    d. Sweep—O_2 L/min.—refers to liters/minute via circuit. CO_2 L/min. refers to carbogen at liters/minute via circuit
    e. ECMO blender FiO_2—amount of fractured-inspired oxygen via circuit
    f. Venous sat—venous saturation in percentage
    g. Arterial sat—arterial saturation in percentage
    h. Preoxygenator and postoxygenator pressures refer to pressure-monitoring procedure
    i. Hemofiltration shunt—see hemofiltration procedure

8. Blood gases.
9. *Medication* refers to name of drug and amount administered in the ECMO circuit document.
10. Fluid therapy.

    a. Heparin—refers to heparin drip and the concentration it is mixed at and the fluid it is mixed in

- Rate/cum.—refers to the rate at which the heparin drip is infusing at over the cumulative balance read at the end of each hour
- Units/kg/hr—refers to the calculated amount of heparin the patient is receiving per kilogram per hour
- ACT—activated clotting time measured in seconds

    b. Unlabeled fluid columns—refers to any IV fluid infusing into the ECMO circuit. To be designated by a letter in the code description column.
    c. FFP, PRBCs, albumin, platelets volume—individual columns refer to blood products infused into the ECMO circuit over the cumulative total infused
    d. Blood products are to be documented in the concurrent blood utilization column.

11. Output

    a. Urine/hr/cum—refers to patient urinary output per hour over cumulative total
    b. Misc./hr/cum—refers to miscellaneous outputs from the ECMO circuit (i.e., hemofiltrate)
    c. Blood out/hr/cum—refers to all blood removed from the ECMO circuit for samples, etc., over the cumulative totals

12. Laboratory results—recorded as written
13. Heparin loading dose—refers to heparin given precannulation written as units per kg
14. Maximum flow rate—refers to calculated flow rate of patient, written as cc's per kilogram
15. Emergency vent. Settings—recorded as written, refers to ventilator settings to be used in case of circuit emergency

IV Fluids

It is preferable to convert IV fluids except those used to maintain pressure-monitoring lines to the pump circuit upon bypass. All IV tubings are to be changed as per unit policy. All peripheral IV sites should be normal saline flushed every four hours. No heparin is required. Should an IV site become infiltrated while on bypass, *do not remove it*. Label it as infiltrated to be removed post-ECMO.

1. **Daily**

    a. All fluids given via patient and circuit will be totaled.
    b. Blood out column will be designated as blood drawn from the patient.
    c. Communicate all laboratory results to MD on call and execute any written orders.
    d. Medications given via the circuit will be charted as per policy.
    e. Weights and head circumference QD or q12 hourly.
    f. Narrative notes that the ECMO specialist or perfusionist is maintaining the ECMO circuit.
    g. Cannula site integrity.

2. **Dressing Changes**

Dressing changes are to be performed as per hospital policy for all central lines. Cannula site dressings are to be changed every twenty-four hours. Strict sterile technique is to be used. The central line dressing kit is well designed for this procedure.

The ECMO specialist should assist the nurse for this procedure. The old dressing is removed and saved to measure any blood loss. The site is cleansed using the Betadine swabs followed by the alcohol swabs. Special care is taken not to remove any formed clots as removal may cause excessive bleeding. Betadine ointment is applied along the suture site, and sterile four by fours are used with clear plastic tape or Tegaderm to form an occlusive site. Documentation should include color, swelling noted, and amount, if any, of bleeding.

While a minimal amount of oozing at the cannulation site is normal, any significant blood loss should be quantitated and replaced, and measures to stop the bleeding should be employed. Gelfoam band thrombin applied directly to the site are recommended. Excessive bleeding may require wound reexploration by the cannulating surgeon.

3. **Emergency Situations**

Caution must be exercised at all times to avoid inadvertent decannulation whenever moving the baby or changing the cannula site dressing. Should accidental decannulation occur, apply direct pressure to just below the incision site, call for help, and institute the emergency ventilator settings. Notify the surgeon for recannulation. Initiation of emergency cardiac support may be necessary.

4. **Special Considerations**

Several factors to take into consideration when a patient is on ECMO:

Sepsis

Sepsis is a concern for ECMO patients. Scrupulous sterile technique must be employed at all times when opening the system. Broad-spectrum antibiotics may be given on a routine basis as a preventive measure. Stopcocks are kept capped and changed every twelve hours. If using vancomycin, it must be given through a nonheparinized line as heparin deactivates vancomycin. Consider plasmapheresis for any patient who has recalcitrant sepsis.

Lungs

It is important during extracorporeal support to recognize that the ECMO circuit, not the ventilator, is maintaining the baby's blood gases. The ventilator is set at minimum levels to allow the lungs to "rest" and prevent the development of ventilator-associated complications such as barotrauma, pneumothorax, and oxygen toxicity. Of equal importance is that ECMO merely "rests" the lungs and cannot cure or treat the disease process. Therefore, the importance of good pulmonary care for the patient on ECMO cannot be overstressed. Postural percussion (vibration only) and drainage should be done periodically, followed by tracheal lavage and suctioning. The patient should also be turned side to side every two hours. Because the baby is completely supported by the ECMO circuit, giving vigorous pulmonary care is easily accomplished. This support allows removal from the ventilator without consequence, for example, to change the endotracheal tube. The patient is heparinized; suctioning by using the measured suctioning technique is required and no nasal suctioning. The use of surfactant may be considered in any patient who has exhibited a deficiency in surfactant. The administration of surfactant should be avoided in patients actively bleeding and is contraindicated with pulmonary hemorrhage.

Central Nervous System (CNS)

The major complications in the neonatal ECMO patient have been CNS related: either cerebral edema or intracranial hemorrhage. CNS problems seem to be related to pre-ECMO levels of hypoxia, acidosis, and/or hypercarbia. Accordingly, neurological checks should be incorporated into the routine care. Included in the neurological check are fontanel tension, pupil size and reaction, level of consciousness, reflexes, and movement. Careful observation of any seizure activity is important as a small focal seizure requires prompt treatment. Phenobarbital has been shown to be effective in the ECMO patient. The baby should be managed under the paralysis protocol with partial or limited paralysis. This should be minimized as the child improves to allow spontaneous respiration.

Renal

Babies on ECMO have Foley catheters placed usually before cannulation. If a catheter is not placed, the baby should be bagged for urine collection to ensure that an accurate output is taken. A low urine output before ECMO is often improved when good perfusion has been achieved on ECMO. Conversely, persistent low urine output may be indicative if poor peripheral perfusion may be associated with a PDA. Acute tubular necrosis is a rare complication in neonatal ECMO patients and most often is a result of the hypotension accompanying the hypoxic state prior to ECMO. Babies who have received massive intravenous fluids secondary to shock or resuscitation are typically very fluid overloaded when placed on ECMO. In addition, sepsis, hypoxia, and ischemia precipitate severe third spacing. These infants are candidates for early hemofiltration. Hemofiltration is used as a last resort when diuretics have failed.

ECMO Specialist Responsibilities

Taking Report

Upon entering the PICU for a scheduled ECMO case, the ECMO specialist first completes a two-minute scrub as per protocol. Report may then be given from the off-going specialist. The following is a standardized guideline for information required during report:

1. Name of patient, age, or DOB
2. History
3. Diagnosis
4. Trends and patterns over the last twenty-four hours
5. Orders, pending medications, and other procedures anticipated for the upcoming shift
6. Any changes or modifications of the current circuit
7. Blood product availability
8. Labs actively pending or needed

Nursing Responsibilities

The nursing care plan should be individualized for each patient on ECMO. There are, however, some responsibilities that are similar for all ECMO patients.

1. Routine hourly vital signs (temp, HR, B/P, CVP).
2. Complete patient assessment q2 hours. Emergency ventilator settings should be noted in red on the ventilator.
3. Strictly measure intake and output q1 hour.
4. Do daily or q12 hourly weights.
5. Assist technician in daily or PRN dressing changes to cannula site.
6. Assist technician in x-rays, ultrasounds, etc.
7. All medications should be administered as per unit policy to the patient. If a medication is to be administered via the pump, the ECMO specialist will prepare it and sign for it.
8. Turn patient q2 hours with assistance of ECMO specialist if the cannulae are stable.
9. DO NOT perform heel sticks, restart peripheral IVs, or administer IM medications. The patient is heparinized.
10. DO NOT suction nasally. Once on bypass, do not insert any nasopharynx tubes.
11. When suctioning endotracheally, use the measured suctioning technique, preferably utilizing two allied health professionals.
12. Every twelve hours, measure head circumference with assistance of ECMO specialist.

ECMO Circuit Checklist

Once a thorough report has been given, an ECMO checklist should be completed.

- Inspection of the circuit from the venous cannula site through the arterial cannula site.
- Touching each connection and fitting, ensuring all are tight connections, identifying each Luer fitting; IV solution and component is important.
- The raceway, if utilized, and bladder should be inspected for excessive wear and clots.
- The sample and infusion sites should be inspected for cracked stopcocks.

- The oxygenator and heat exchanger should be checked for air bubbles or clots.
- Tracing the circuit from the venous to arterial side identifies any circuit modification.
- Tie bands should be applied to any connection in which a connector has been added.

Restocking the ECMO Cart

The ECMO cart should be restocked according to the content list at the end of each off-going shift. Necessary disposable items should be readily available (syringes, saline, ACT tubes). The pump cart and circuit should also be clean and tidy. All spills should be immediately cleaned and sanitized. The ECMO specialist on pump at decannulation is responsible for properly restocking, cleaning, and returning cart to storage area.

Blood Product Availability

It is the responsibility of each ECMO specialist to ensure that all required blood products are available at the start of each shift. If not, orders for blood products needed are sent via computer to the blood bank.

Blood Refrigerator

ECMO specialist must check blood availability with the blood bank and blood refrigerator located in the unit every change of shift. The temperature must be marked as noted (1°C-5°C). The blood refrigerator temperature has to be checked daily. This documentation must be recorded daily. It is the responsibility of the specialist to assure this is done. Once the ECMO case is complete, the blood must be returned to the blood bank.

Blood Bank Policy

It is the responsibility of each ECMO specialist to ensure that all blood product slips are returned to the blood bank at the end of every shift.

Fluid and Medication Administration

Any IV fluid may be administered into the circuit if there is limited patient IV access. The following standards are in effect:

1. All IVF must be on an autosyringe or infusion pump.
2. All IVF must be administered prebladder.
3. All lines are to have a microbubble air detector in line.
4. All pigtails through which an IVF may be infusing must be checked every shift for air, clots, or sediment. If either is present, it must be aspirated, discarded, and the line flushed clear.

5. Any medication may be administered into the circuit if patient access is limited.

   a. All medications must be administered prebladder. **EXCEPTIONS**: lipids or drugs made with or containing fat emulsions are to be given **postoxygenator** through a peripheral line.
   b. The pigtail must be flushed clear when complete.
   c. The medication must be signed off and documented.

Special Procedures during ECMO

Blood Sampling from Circuit

1. Withdraw 0.4 mL "waste" blood. Always discard the "waste" blood when aspirating a sample; *do not reinfuse*.
2. Never inject into the system without aspirating any air bubbles that may be in the stopcock. (If adding an IV line, first fill the stopcock with flush solution then make an airless connection.)
3. Always leave every stopcock capped, either with a sterile syringe or cap.

Changing Stopcocks

1. Always use Luer lock stopcocks.
2. Change frequently used or sticky stopcocks on a PRN basis.
3. Prepare a new stopcock by adding a syringe filled with flush solution and expelling all air from the stopcock.
4. Turn to *off* the most proximal stopcock.
5. Unscrew the stopcock to be changed and discard.
6. Add the new stopcock, aspirate to remove any air, and turn to *off* position.

Ultrasound / Echocardiogram

Ultrasounds are performed daily on all neonates to assess for intraventricular hemorrhage (IVH). This procedure requires the assistance of the ECMO specialist. It is the responsibility of the specialist to maintain the integrity of the cannulas to avoid inadvertent bumping or moving of the cannulas where accidental decannulation may occur.

Surgical Intervention

In some instances, surgical intervention may be necessary while on bypass. It is recommended that most surgical procedures be performed in the pediatric intensive care unit. These procedures include PDA ligations, thoracotomies, diaphragm repairs, and laparotomies and all procedures involving cannulae placement. Only for most complicated procedures should the patient be transported to the operating room on ECMO. Once the decision for surgery has been made, the specialist will need to make certain changes in management.

Apheresis Utilizing the ECMO Circuit

Apheresis is indicated when a clinical need to separate blood components arises from a patient's medical condition. These separated components may be exchanged, depleted, or collected for transfusion at a later date. Apheresis pulls and returns at the same rate, so ECLS flow will not be affected.

Responsibilities

1. Verify procedure with apheresis specialist.
2. Assist apheresis specialist to explain rationale and procedure to family.
3. Record patient height and weight.
4. Send baseline preprocedure labs CBC, Ica^{++}, and P8 (notify physician of results).
5. Extra labs only for specific procedures (notify physician of results).
   a. TSM (red cell exchange)
   b. Need HIV consent first
   c. Need consent for stem cell
   d. CD34 and disease markers
6. Extra labs for multiple procedures (notify physician of results).
   a. Mg and PO_4
   b. PT/PTT

c. FDP, fibrinogen if ordered
7. Standby emergency replacement fluid (PRBCs, albumin, FFP, NS).
8. Connect apheresis access line (using sterile and airless technique) to venous pigtail close to patient (preoxygenator).
9. Connect apheresis return line (using sterile and airless technique) to any of the venous pigtails downstream from access line and preoxygenator (prebladder).
10. Halfway through procedure or if symptomatic for hypocalcaemia, send ICa (notify physician of results).
11. Monitor ACTs; apheresis uses citrate to bond calcium to prevent clotting; adjustments in heparin may be necessary.
12. If patient deteriorates, stop apheresis run, notify physician STAT, and follow ECLS protocol.
13. When it's completed, disconnect apheresis access and return line (using sterile and airless technique) and flush pigtails with 1 cc NS and place port cap on site.
14. Postprocedure: send ICa, P8, and PT/PTT (notify physician of results).

The ECMO specialist can easily perform therapeutic apheresis, total plasma exchange, red blood cell exchange, leukopheresis, and stem cell collection. Blood is withdrawn through a stopcock on the venous line and returned downstream on the venous line. Venous drainage from the patient is not affect, and this will not affect venous blood flow through the ECMO circuit. Standard apheresis protocols from the manufacturer should be followed.

Hemofiltration

In cases of low urine output and/or hypervolemia, hemofiltration may be undertaken to maintain intake and output balance. Only after a PDA has been ruled out and other aggressive management techniques have failed (diuretics) should hemofiltration be considered. The ECMO circuit easily facilitates it as it provides easy blood access. The patient is already systemically heparinized; no further anticoagulation is needed in the dialysis circuit. The manufacturer recommends the use of the hemofilter for short periods of time. The hemofilter will be changed every twenty-four hours if extended filtration is required. If the patient requires dialysis, then hemodiafiltration may be set up, according to the dialysis orders provided.

Materials and Equipment

1. Transonic flowmeter on patient arterial cannula
2. One (1) 500 c bag NS
3. One (1) albumin IV line
4. One (1) Minifilter Plus (hemofilter)
5. Three (3) three-way stopcocks
6. Two (2) green tubing clamps
7. Three (3 [4 if dialysis]) 33" IV extension tubing
8. One (1) IV pump
9. One (1) half-set IV tubing
10. One (1) urimeter

Hemofilter/Tubing Assembly

Maintaining sterile technique

1. Don proper personal protection equipment (PPE), including surgical hat, mask, and gloves when assembling sterile equipment and tubing pack.
2. Connect three-way stopcocks to male ends of two 33" IV extension tubing (one venous, one arterial).
3. Connect female ends of 33" IV extension tubing to top and bottom ports of Minifilter (venous, arterial); close stopcocks both ends.
4. Connect three-way stopcock to female end of one 33" IV extension tubing of the ultra filtration line, two if performing dialysis.
5. Connect male end of 33" IV extension tubing to side port of Minifilter, venous end.
6. Leave white cap on arterial side port (used to add dialysate).

Priming Hemofilter

7. Spike albumin IV tubing to bag of heparinized saline.
8. Connect heparinized saline to stopcock on arterial tubing.
9. Clamp Minifilter side port tubing.
10. Hold filter vertical red arrow facing up (venous port).
11. Prime internal portion of filter (blood path) with heparinized saline from arterial to venous side, tapping filter to remove air.
12. When 2/3 bag used in prime, clamp off venous line and prime bag (arterial side remains open at this time).
13. Open clamp on hemofilter side port tubing.

14. Keeping filter on vertical position (red arrow facing up open), prime outside of filter (filter will slowly fill from bottom up).
15. When prime exits hemofiltration port and tubing, clamp off arterial line and hemofiltration lines (arterial, venous, and hemofiltration lines should be clamped); you are ready to attach to ultrafiltration circuit.

Connecting Filter to Ultrafiltration Circuit

16. Place male/male connector on end of 33" IV extension tubing (side port of Minifilter).
17. Connect male/male connector to primed ½ set in IV pump.
18. Connect end of IV tubing ¼ male Luer.
19. Cut off connector to Urimeter tubing and place ¼ end from ¼ male connector into urimeter tubing.
20. Once filter is connected to ECMO circuit, IV pump will be set to draw off ultrafiltrate as per MD orders.

Connecting Filter to ECMO Circuit

21. Connect arterial (access) tubing on hemofilter to postpump-preoxygenator pigtail.
22. Connect venous (return) tubing to prebladder pigtail.
23. Tape Minifilter to support bar on ECMO circuit.
24. Open arterial then venous clamps, adjusting ECMO flow to maintain transonic flow to patient.
25. Open clamp on ultrafiltration line and set IV pump to pull off desired amount of ultrafiltrate.

Ultrafiltrate Removal

26. An order for total filtrate to remove per hour is received from the physician.
27. Connect the distal end of the ultrafiltrate tubing to the spike of an infusion set (the ultrafiltrate line represents the IV bag).
28. An infusion rate is set by the pump and will be the allowed ultrafiltration rate prescribed.
29. This infusion pump at the prescribed flow rate removes ultrafiltrate slowly.
30. Monitor the patient's vital signs for hypervolemia, electrolyte changes, and decreasing heparin levels.

31. If intermittent filtration is ordered, once the correct amount of filtrate is removed or when there is deterioration in vital signs, the ultrafiltrate tubing is clamped and the pump turned off. For continuous filtration, monitor hourly.

Special Consideration for Hemofiltration

32. The removal of the total amount of filtrate will be spaced evenly over the hour.
33. At the end of the hour, the total amount removed should be documented on the ECMO flow sheet as output.
34. While the hemofilter is in the ECMO circuit, the total flow display is not accurate for what the patient is receiving.
35. The use of a specific flowmeter is important to measure the accurate flow going to the ECMO patient.
36. It is estimated that approximately 100-150 mL/min. of flow is diverted through the hemofilter (even when partially occluded). Because of this, weaning the flow while the hemofilter is in line is inaccurate.
37. The specialist must remember to maintain flows higher than the 100 mL/min. for idling. The baby may actually be at idling speed when the flow display is at 200 mL/min.
38. It is generally recommended that if active weaning is going to take place, the hemofilter should be removed.
39. Careful observance of the ACTs should be a priority when the specialist is actively hemofiltering. Because of the hemofilter's filtering system, heparin is removed along with various electrolytes and free water. Therefore, the heparin consumption may increase per hour.
40. Careful intake and output balances must be maintained. The infant's insensible water losses must also be taken into consideration. It is recommended that a cumulative intake and output from the beginning of the case be kept. This gives a much more accurate assessment of the baby's current balance.
41. Daily weights should also be done at a regular time each day or every twelve hours if required.

Measuring Preoxygenator and Postoxygenator Pressures with Hemofiltration

The altering of cerebral blood flow with ECMO has been well documented. The following protocol will decrease accidental hyperperfusion to the cerebral vessels.

1. Note the Transonic blood flow rate in "normal" conditions (hemofilter blood flow open).
2. Decrease the ECMO pump flow rate until it matches the value in number.
3. Quickly turn off the blood flow to the hemofilter. One one-way stopcock anywhere in the hemofilter circuit will adequately perform this function.
4. Look at the Transonic flowmeter and note that the flow equals value in number 1.
5. If it does not match this value, adjust the pump until the Transonic flow rate equals the value in number 1.
6. Once this adjustment is made, recalibrate the jostra "flow" display until the value matches the value on the Transonic flowmeter.
7. Measure preoxygenator and postoxygenator pressures per protocol.
8. Reopen the hemofilter blood flow.
9. Increase the ECMO flow rate until the Transonic flowmeter matches the flow rate in value number 1.
10. Recalculate hemofilter flow rate and document.
11. If recalibration of the ECMO pump flow rate display was performed, note *Recall* on the flow sheet and the progress notes.

CAVH-D Continuous Arterial Venous Hemodiafiltration

A. Dialysis

- When a patient needs hemodialysis, despite hemofiltration, it is necessary to dialyze the patient's blood.
- An additional pump is set up to deliver dialysis fluid (Dianeal) to the second ultrafiltrate outlet of the hemofilter.
- An additional pump controls the ultrafiltrate outlet pressure; thus, the amount of actual fluid removed.
- The volume infused should be at the maximum infusion rate minus the amount of diuresis required.
    o For example, inflow is set at 900 mL/min; the outflow is set at 960 mL/min. Fluid removal will be at 60 mL.
- Electrolyte stability and removal is dependent on the chemical composition of the dialysate.
- Dialysate is prescribed in conjunction with the measured renal requirements.

B. Indications for Hemodiafiltration/Dialysis

1. Renal failure or electrolyte disturbances for any of the following:

   a. Na > 165
   b. K > 6.0
   c. BUN > 90
   d. Creatinine > 2.5
   e. Metabolic acidosis pH < 7.20

2. Any Neurologic abnormality secondary to uremia, electrolyte disturbances secondary to Ca^{++}, PO_4
3. Removal of any toxic substance with dialysis or charcoal perfusion

IN VIVO OCCLUSION SETTING PROTOCOL

A. Shopping List

- (1) two-foot-long PVC monitoring line
- Stopcock
- Sodium chloride
- 60 mL syringe
- 6 mL syringe

B. Procedure

1. Preprime monitor line with sodium chloride.
2. Attach a two-foot monitor line with stopcock and 6 mL syringe to ACT sample port.
3. Aspirate air from monitor line.
4. Close stopcock.
5. Connect 60 mL syringe to bladder port.
6. Come off bypass, pump, then vein-bridge-artery.
7. Emergency ventilator settings.
8. Clamp preoxygenator; post ACT sample site.
9. Clamp prebladder.
10. Set both rollers per diagram.
11. Totally occlude tubing with roller thumb wheel.
12. Withdraw blood/fluid into the 60 mL syringe until the bladder box alarms.
13. Silence alarms.

14. Hold stopcock and monitor line level with the top of the oxygenator.
15. Open stopcock on top of the monitor line.
16. Watch column of fluid in monitor line; it should not move.
17. Deocclude raceway one click at a time, watching for fluid column to fall on monitor line.
18. Deocclude until fluid movement is consistent (no stopping).
19. Close stopcock on top of the monitor line.
20. Turn off the ACT sample site.
21. Remove the two-foot monitor line.
22. Reinfuse the volume in the 60 mL syringe back into bladder.
23. Remove prebladder clamp.
24. Remove preoxygenator clamp.
25. Circuit check.
26. Go back on bypass per protocol, artery-bridge-vein.
27. Turn alarms back on Seabrook bladder controller.

Transporting a Patient on ECMO

1. Notify perfusionist, priming specialist, ECMO coordinator, and designee fellow.
2. Check battery for charge status.
3. Notify respiratory care for *E* cylinder of oxygen with regulator and flowmeter.
4. Convert all IV pumps to portable; attach several to ECMO cart if necessary.
5. Obtain pretransport blood gas; document results before transport. Draw up large syringes (60 mL) of albumin and normal saline for emergencies.
6. Once patient is ready to transport, ECMO preparation includes the following:
    a. Change sweep to *E* cylinder at the same oxygen flow rate.
    b. Quickly transfer power cord from bladder controller to the battery plugged into wall.
7. Assess proper pump function.
8. Acquire power cord from maintenance, umbilical line from unit to the OR for standby use.
9. Unplug SVO2 and move to base of warmer.
10. Unplug ACT machine and place in base of warmer.
11. Plug water heater CSZ into outlet on the battery supply.

12. When the battery is unplugged, immediately turn off the water heater as this component is the highest energy consumer in the ECMO system.
13. If transporting on radiant warmer bed, turn up temperature of overhead warmer.
14. When ready to transport, the ECMO specialist (CES) will hold the baby's catheters in one hand and the ECMO bed in the other, acting as an anchor for the cannula to the bed.
15. The CES will give all directional orders. If *anyone* assisting with the transport says *stop*, all will immediately stop, and whatever problem is occurring will be assessed and resolved. When the CES assesses that all is stable, the transport will continue with the CES managing all movements of bed and pump.
16. Once stable in the destination, the battery should immediately be plugged into an emergency outlet.
17. Turn on water heater after battery is plugged into the wall; turn down radiant warmer temperature.
18. Once the procedure is concluded, assess portability of all devices, pumps, and bed.
19. Repeat steps 7 and 8 above.
20. Once stabilized in the bed space, all devices should be plugged into emergency outlets.
21. Return the battery to standby.
22. Plug the battery into a wall outlet and verify charging status.

Chapter 6

Hematologic Considerations on ECMO

Newborn Considerations[35, 36]

Birth being the moment of maximum life places extraordinary challenges on the infants who require ECMO. These factors are by definition overwhelming, and below is a partial list:

- Common neonatal ECMO pathophysiology
  - Hypoxia, ischemia
  - Hypotension
  - Hypothermia
  - Acidosis
  - Infection
  - Hepatic dysfunction
  - Renal failure
  - Hypoglycemia
  - Hypocalcaemia
  - Hypomagnesaemia
  - Anemia
  - Thrombocytopenia
  - DIC

The structure for understanding coagulation was first provided by Virchow in 1858.[34] The triad, in addition to the above factors, to understanding the hematology, coagulation, thrombosis, and hemorrhage of the ECMO patient are the following:[35, 36]

- Vascular system
- Blood flow / stasis
- Coagulation cofactors

Vascular System

- The ECMO circuit is a prosthetic, negatively charged, nonhomogeneous, surface area that equals, in some cases, twice the circulating blood volume of the newborn. The thrombogenicity of the surface has been related to the activation and adherence of fibrinogen.
- This negatively charged surface stimulates factor XII, thromboxane B_2, fibrinogen, compliment, and platelets.
- There is a direct endothelial injury associated with ECMO. The exposure leads to constant surface activation, activation of the thromboplastic cascade, and increased thrombosis. The common pathophysiology factors listed above exaggerate the cascade.

Blood Flow / Stasis

- Regional changes in blood flow during bypass lead to alterations of laminar and turbulent areas. Stagnant areas of flow in addition to common pathophysiology contribute to increased thrombosis.
- Poor peripheral blood flow, nonpulsatile blood flow add to thrombosis.
- Red cell blood cell stress from the cyclical loading of shear stress during pump occlusion can be measured by the index of hemolysis. This relates the efficiency of the pump flow with the release of free hemoglobin over time. Newton's shear equation and Reynolds's turbulent shear equation may both be used to directly measure cyclic loading.[37]

Coagulation Cofactors

1. **Normal newborn coagulation** is a balance from birth. A newborn exhibits a *serum measured cofactor partial hypocoagulable state* to deal with birthing.

- An increased aPTT secondary to decreased factors XII and XI, prekallikrein, and HMW Kininogen
- An increased PT secondary to a decrease in vitamin K, factors II, VII, IX, and X
- An increase in thomboplastin time (TT) from decreased fibrinogen

2. **The stressed newborn** exhibits a *whole-blood measured hypercoagulability*.

- A decrease in bleeding time due to
  o Hyperviscosity and increased von Willebrand factor.
- A decreased ACT secondary to
  o Decreased plasminogen
  o Increased clot resistance to fibrinolysis
  o A decrease in factors II, V, and VII also play a part
- Relative deficiencies of protein S and protein C.
- Increased platelet aggregation and thrombosis secondary to
  o Hypoxia, which releases vasoactive adenosine diphosphate (ADP), epinephrine, and thromboxane A_2

3. **The infant placed on ECMO** may receive up to a one-to-two-time blood volume transfusion in the first few days.

- Massive transfusions lead to a decrease in 2, 3, DPG, platelet count and function, hypocalcaemia, hypoglycemia, acidosis, citrate toxicity, hypothermia, hyperkalemia, and microembolization.
- A further dilutional decrease in factors II, V, and VII and platelets.
- See above list of risk factors.

Clot Formation

Two types of clots are commonly encountered by ecmologists.

- A true clot is referring to the formation and deposition of fibrin with the stimulation and trapping of platelets, red blood cells, and white blood cells.
- This is a fully organized and structurally and chemically active clot that leads to thrombosis, physical clotting, and embolization.
- A true clot will not be formed in areas of high laminar flow.
- A white clot or fibrin clot may be formed in areas of laminar flow with the transient aggregation of platelets and white blood cells. This is often a transient phenomenon.

Passive Therapy

Nonpharmaceutical management of coagulation involves managing the ECMO flow and the design of the ECMO circuit.

ECMO Flow—Higher ECMO flows

- Reduce stasis
- Increases laminar flow, which
    - Increases the natural release of tissue plasminogen factor (TPA)
    - Reduces the quantitative need for systemic anticoagulation (heparin)
    - Heparin infusion can be stopped during high-flow ECMO conditions with cautious monitoring of ACTs

ECMO Circuit

- This guide strongly recommends maintaining the practice of protein priming all circuits during the setup.
- Significant strides have been made to primarily bind protein molecules to the internal surface of the entire ECMO circuit. By and large, it is relatively easy to acquire a completely coated surface.
- These surfaces significantly reduce the negatively charged stimulation of cofactors.
- Unfortunately, they also bind molecules, and some have a strong tendency to bind ATIII.
- There is a reduction in circulating ATII levels and heparin effect.

Chapter 7

Blood Product Administration

Blood products may be administered into the ECMO circuit safely premembrane or postmembrane (except platelets are postmembrane only). Proper filters must be used. Caution must take place to avoid injection of air. All blood products that are transfused, including those directly to the patient, must be documented on the concurrent blood utilization section of the ECMO flow sheet. The donor number and justification for administration of the product must be written. Types of blood products are discussed here.

Packed Red Blood Cells (PRBCs)

PRBCs may be administered into the circuit via a prebladder pigtail. In emergency situations, they may be administered directly with a Luer lock syringe. In cases of transfusion over an hour or more, an autosyringe or infusion pump setup should be used. Once the transfusion is complete, the access port is flushed with sterile saline and capped.

PRBCs may be administered in the following instances to the following:

   a. Prime the ECMO circuit
   b. Maintain the hemoglobin 12-15 Hgb
   c. Maintain the hematocrit 35-45 Hct
   d. Maintain central venous pressure greater than 5 as a volume replacement if indicated by Hgb / Hct
   e. Maintain mean arterial pressure within age indicated ranges as volume replacement as indicated by Hgb / Hct

f. Replace patient blood loss due to lab sampling or hemorrhage or circuit emergency
g. Replace volume for hypovolemia if indicated by Hgb / Hct for pumps "chattering"
h. Increase oxygen delivery by ability to increase pump flow to maintain physiologic needs in unstable patients, increase hemoglobin content
i. Increase peripheral vascular resistance

Fresh Frozen Plasma (FFP)

FFP is administered in the same manner as PRBCs. It may be given in the following instances:

a. Priming the ECMO circuit
b. Maintaining central venous pressure greater than 5 as a volume replacement if indicated by Hgb / Hct
c. Volume replacement for hypovolemia with PRBCs in ratio of 1 FFP to 3 PRBCs
d. Uncontrollable hemorrhage a ratio of 1 FFP to 1 PRBC
e. Persistent increase in activated clotting times (ACTs) with an increase in total units/kg/hr heparin administration
f. Deficiency of antithrombin III (ATIII)
g. Heparin administration less than 10 units/kg/hr (evidence of DIC)
h. Persistent decreases in ACTs with an increase in heparin units/kg/hr
i. Low heparin levels from increased excretion or immunologic intolerance
j. Massive transfusion reaction
k. Clinical or laboratory suspicion of infection or sepsis, immune deficiencies, undefined coagulopathy, or hypoproteinemia

Platelets

Platelets must *only* be given through a peripheral venous line or when necessary *postoxygenator*. An access port with double stopcocks is positioned on the Y for this purpose. The access port is debubbled first, and only 10-20 mL Luer tip syringes are to be used. Platelets may be given directly to the patient if they are pooled or superpacked. Once the transfusion is complete, the access port is flushed with sterile saline.

- The platelet level should be maintained high, greater than one hundred thousand if possible.

- This may be achieved by transfusing one or more superpack of platelets (seven units of pooled platelets).
- *Aprotinin* (a kallekrein inhibitor) may improve platelet function if bleeding is a problem.
- Von Willibrand factor must be measured if platelet pathology is suspected.
- Changes in source of heparin will affect platelets.
- Maternal or acquired (autoimmune) antibodies must be evaluated during platelets' pathology.
- Alterations of the circuit with the introduction, replacement, or removal of devices, tubing, or equipment will alter platelets.
- Circuit coating will alter platelet function.
- Vasopressin (DDAVP) through the stimulation of von Willibrand factor will improve platelets activity.
- Heparin-induced thrombotic thrombocytopenia (HIT).

  o This is an autoimmune disorder.
  o Multiple white arterial thrombi are present with a platelet count less than ten thousand in spite of repeated platelet transfusion.
  o Changing the source of heparin may help this problem.
  o Apheresis is a consideration.
  o Alternative anticoagulation therapies such as argatroban.

The infusion of platelets and occasionally cryoprecipitate is a necessary procedure during ECLS. Present ECLS technology describes an extreme thrombocytopenia related to extracorporeal circulation, particularly when using the silicone membrane oxygenator for gas exchange. The purpose of this protocol is to ease the complexity of this procedure and ensure stability in patient oxygenation and coagulation status.

1. Obtain platelets or cryoprecipitate from the blood bank (crossmatched).
2. After checking the blood, draw the platelets into a 60 mL syringe using a 20-micron blood/platelet filter.
3. Connect a 36" IV extension tubing to the syringe.
4. Dabble the line by infusing the platelets.
5. Connect the monitor line to the platelet infusion port (postoxygenator).
6. Note the remaining volume in the syringe and set the infusion rate to the same. The platelets will be infused over fifteen minutes.
7. Double the continuous heparin infusion.

8. Start the infusion of platelets into the circuit.
9. Monitor ACTs q15" or PRN.
10. Gradual increases and decreases in heparin infusion are recommended. Ten percent changes in this rate should compensate for minimal changes in the ACT. Without the doubling of the heparin infusion, platelet infusion can/will dangerously lower the patient's ACT.
11. Perform an ACT prior to any administration.

    a. If ACT is > 200 seconds, give 10 mL. Repeat ACT within fifteen minutes.
    b. If ACT is 180-200 seconds, give ten units heparin bolus, give 10 mL, repeat ACT.
    c. If ACT is 170-180 seconds, give twenty units heparin bolus, give 10 mL, repeat ACT.
    d. If ACT is < 160 seconds, give twenty to thirty units heparin bolus, repeat ACT until within desired range.

12. ACTs should be repeated every fifteen minutes, and adjustment of the heparin drip may be required to maintain ACTs in the desired range. Doubling the heparin infusion dose during platelets administration will maintain ACTs within desired range. The bridge must remain clamped during infusion. **Do not** flash bridge. Previous therapeutic heparin dose can be resumed postinfusion with ACTs monitored every fifteen minutes for at least thirty minutes.

13. Maintain ordered parameters during administration. Transfusion may need to be slowed (5 mL every fifteen minutes) if difficulties arise. Platelets may be administered in the following instances:
    a. To maintain a platelet count greater than one hundred thousand
    b. Uncontrollable hemorrhage
        a. When the platelet count is desired to be at a higher level, such as in the case of IVH or elective surgical procedure

Calcium—ionized calcium levels must be maintained above 1.0 mg/dl.

Magnesium—magnesium levels must be maintained above 2.0mg/dl.

Cryoprecipitate

The administration of cryoprecipitate into the ECMO circuit is not recommended. If physician orders and patient status merit such use, the recommendation is to give via a peripheral IV directly to the patient and monitor ACTs accordingly unless no other access is available.

Cryoprecipitate may be administered in the following instances:

- If the fibrinogen level is less than 200 mg/dl
- If the fibrin split products are greater than 40 mg/dl
- Uncontrollable hemorrhage (fibrin glue)

Albumin (5%)

Albumin is to be administered in the same manner as PRBCs for emergencies or volume replacement when the patient's hemoglobin/hematocrit coagulation is within normal limits. Albumin may be administered in the following instances:

a. As volume replacement for hypovolemia when Hgb / Hct are within normal parameters or when awaiting PRBCs
b. Maintain central venous pressure greater than five as indicated by Hgb / Hct
c. Maintain mean arterial pressure as indicated by Hgb / Hct
d. Maintain colloid oncotic pressure
e. Evidence of hypoproteinemia or ongoing protein losses
g. Unavailability of FFP
h. To decrease peripheral vascular resistance

Albumin (25 %)

Albumin is to be administered in the same manner as PRBCs. It is to be administered in the following instances:

a. For priming the ECMO circuit
b. For clinical or laboratory evidence of severe third spacing
c. Evidence of capillary leak syndrome
d. All instances listed for albumin 5%
e. Plasmalyte is to be administered in the same manner and instances as Albumin 5%

Amicar

Epsilon-aminocaproic acid (Amicar) inhibits the zymogen formation of plasmin from plasminogen. Plasmin is responsible for the breakdown of the fibrin clot. Amicar decreases levels of systemic plasmin, thereby increasing the fibrin clot formation and inhibiting fibrinolysis. This decreases the amount of bleeding, particularly in perioperative patients. Doing a thromboelastograms (TEG) prior to Amicar administration is warranted. When a patient is having a large amount of intrinsic bleeding, despite appropriate levels of platelets and coagulation factors, Amicar may be given to the patient or perioperatively.

The dose is 50-100 mg/kg bolus over one hour then a continuous drip of 10-40 mg/kg/hr.

This drug will help attain homeostasis in the anticoagulated ECLS patient. **It will also precipitate clotting in the extracorporeal circuitry.** Amicar is indicated only for patients at high risk for hemorrhage. This includes all postop patients (i.e., congenital diaphragmatic hernia, postop cardiac repair, etc.) and pediatric and neonatal patients with a grade I intracranial hemorrhage.

Amicar therapy is regulated to maintain the following:

- ACT   160-200 (flow dependent)
- FDP   10-40
- Fibrinogen   > 200
- Platelets   > 150

The ECMO specialist should do as follows:

1. Be very aware of clots in the circuits
2. Closely monitor preoxygenator and postoxygenator pressures
3. Manage the heparin appropriately (ACT as ordered by MD)
4. Maximize attainable blood flow (> 200 cc/min.)
5. Discontinue Amicar if the flow is dropped below two hundred mL/min (200 mL/min)
6. Decrease or discontinue Amicar and have the fellow or attending notified if sudden or excessive clot formation is noted

Alteplase

Recombinant tissue-type plasminogen activator (alteplase) preferentially activates plasminogen bound to fibrin. This creates fibrinolysis that is confirmed to a thrombus, avoiding systemic activation of plasminogen. R-tPA may be administered directly into a blood vessel of a patient on ECMO that becomes acutely and severely occluded and the distal circulation is at severe risk of ischemic.

The initial dose is a bolus of 0.48 mg/ kg followed by an infusion of 0.27 mg/kg/hr for six hours. Careful clinical monitoring of extremity and/ or perfusion and sudden life-threatening bleeding is necessary. Discontinue infusion if any clinical indication of bleeding occurs.

Recombinant Antithrombin III (rATIII)

Thrombate or Atryn—one unit/ kg raise ATIII 1% (1u/mL); the dose is usually 75 units/kg

Heparin-Induced Thrombotic Thrombocytopenia (HIT)

This is an autoimmune disorder that is characterized by multiple white arterial thrombi and a platelet count less than ten thousand in spite of repeated platelet transfusion. Changing the source of heparin may help this problem. Apheresis is a consideration as well as alternative anticoagulation therapies such as **argatroban.** The dose of argatroban is usually 0.75 mcg/kg.min for 2 hours, inc. 0.1 mcg/kg/min until greater than PTT 60.

Fibrin Glue Sealant Preparation and Application

In separate 12 mL syringes, 10 mL of cryoprecipitate (crossmatched with the patient) is drawn into one syringe, and 250 mg of CaC1 (2.5 mL) plus 7.5 mL of thrombin (mixed as per manufacturer's policy) into the other syringe. By simultaneously injecting this solution onto the site, thorough mixing is achieved. This simultaneous mixing is preferred to sequential application because it achieves the greatest tensile strength and resultant immediate hemostasis.

Once the mixture has been applied, the site should be dressed with sterile four by fours and plastic tape. When the dressing is changed, care should be taken not to dislodge the clot. This will interrupt any clotting that may have already taken effect.

If the bleeding is extreme and will not be controlled by the recommended steps, reexploration of the site may be necessary by the cardiovascular surgeon. If hemorrhage is life threatening or surgery is unsuccessful, contraindicated, or worsening bleeding, then the heparin may be turned off. A new circuit may be primed at the bedside and immediately available. Amicar should be turned off, preferably thirty minutes prior. Constant inspection of the circuit for clots is required. The highest flow allowed by the patient is preferred.

Alternative Anticoagulation Therapies

- Ancrod—A serine protease inhibitor derived from pit viper venom
    o Dose 0.8 U/kg/hr for 12 hours then 0.4 U/kg/hr for 60 hours[38]

- Low molecular weight heparin (LMWH)—A depolymerized heparin; the subcutaneous administration limits it application

- Lomoparin—A synthetic organon heparinoid
    o 80% heparin (Dermatan and chondroitin sulfate)
    o May be useful for patients with HIT

- Nafamostat mesilate—A short acting "regional" protease inhibitor
    o Dose: 0.2-0.4 milligram per kilogram per hour[39]

Thromboelastogram (TEG)[40, 41]

Developed in 1948 by Hartert, the TEG is as an automated measurement device that provides details of whole blood activity. The diagram below is a thromboelastogram that represents an in vitro measurement of whole blood clotting.

Thromboelastogram (TEG)

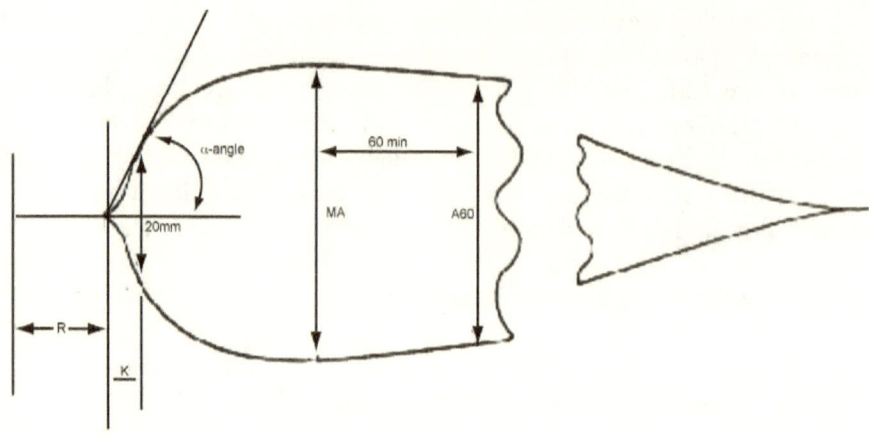

The graph above designates the following variable:

R— Measures clotting time
Relates to the amount of heparin
Increased with hypocoagulability; **treat with FFP (cryo, VIIa)**
Decreased with hypercoagulability
Prolonged with a coagulation factor deficiency

K— Measures clot formation; **treat with cryo (FFP, VIIa)**

α (angle)—Measures kinetics of clot formation; **treat with cryo (FFP, VIIa)**
Decreased with Fibrinogen Deficiency

MA— Reflects Clot Strength; **treat with platelets**
Fibrinolysis
Affect by fibrinogen, platelet count, and function

Ly30— Fibrinolysis activity (Ly60≈A60)

TEG Graphic Representations[40, 41]

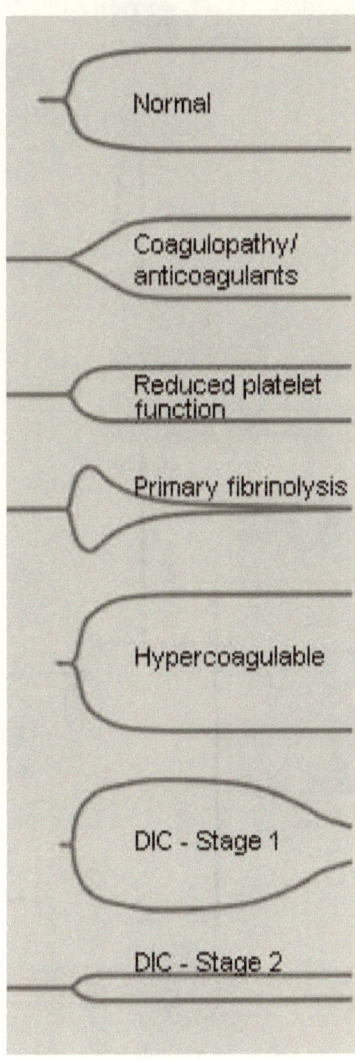

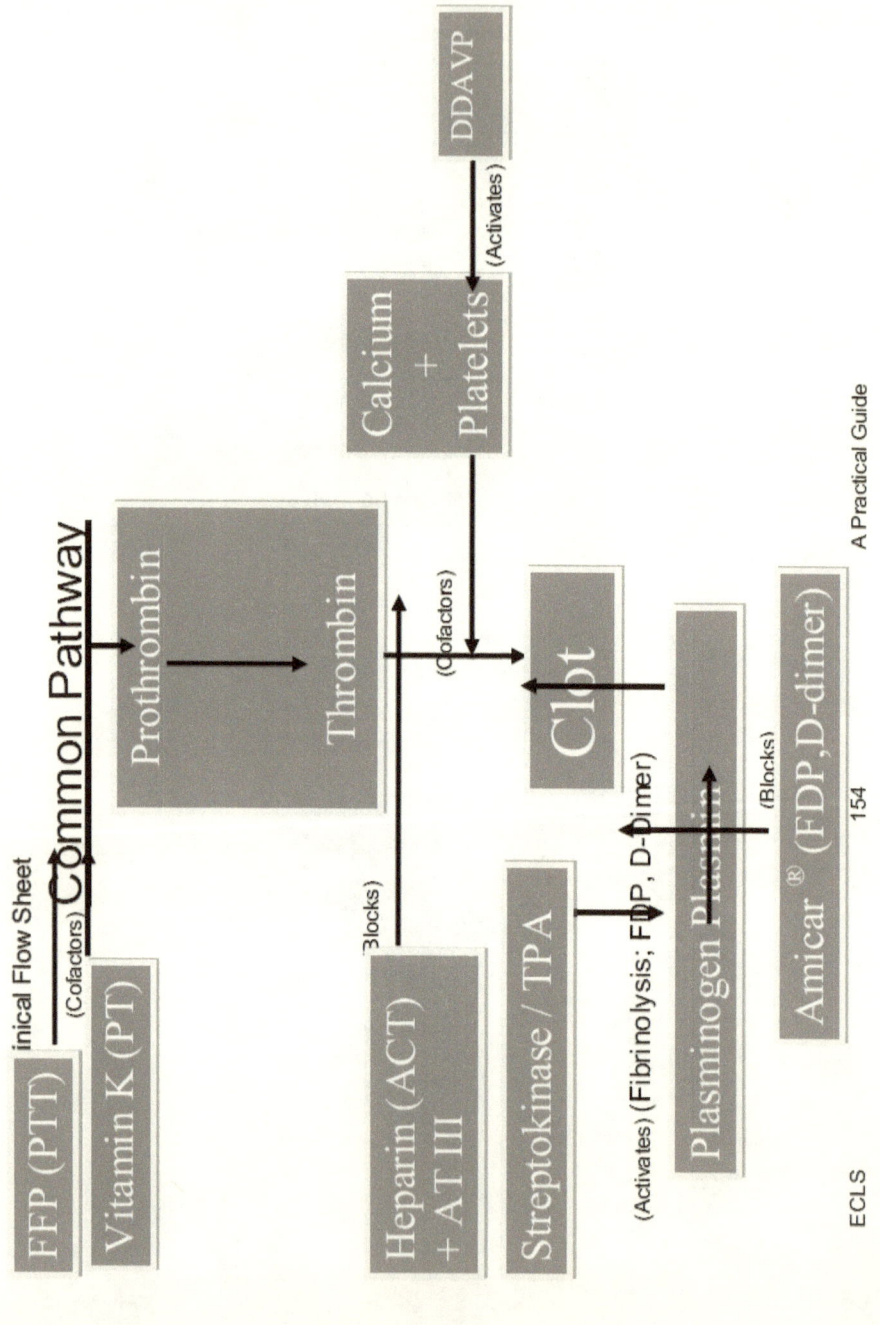

Anticoagulation Quality Management Tool

ECLS Anticoagulation QM Tool							Page 1
Date			Specialist		Patient		MR#
Protocol *	qam	prn	Hep, ACT, ATIII, Anti Xa, PT/PTT, fibrinogen, CBC, platelet, TEG				
	q12h	prn	ATIII, H/H, Platelet				
	q1h	prn	ACT				
*Record hourly levels and intervention							

Worksheet	Range	Time	Value	Intervention	Considerations	*Dose
Heparin (U/kg/hr)	25-50 U/Kg/hr	800			Higher flow lower ACT, lower flow higher ACT	**see protocol
ACT	160-180 sec.				Higher flow lower ACT, lower flow higher ACT	
AT III	60%-100%				Give FFP/ATIII if ACT low and heparin is high	FFP 20 mL/kg, ATIII
Anti Xa	0.25-0.6 IU/mL				Give heparin / ATIII when Anti Xa is low	FFP 10-20 mL/k/ heparin
H/H	Hct 35%-45%				VO_2, CO, SVR	10 mL/kg PRBCs
PT	12-14 sec.				Give vit. K when high	1-3 mg per dose q 12h
PTT	60-90 sec.				Give FFP when high	FFP 10-20 mL/kg
Fibrinogen	150-200 mg/dl				Give cryo when low	1 Unit / 5 Kg.
FDP	< 40mcg/mL				DIC when high (consider FFP, cryo, Amicar)	
Platelet Count	> 80,000				> 100,000 for bypass initiation then > 80,000	< 10 Kg— 10 mL/kg
Thromboelastogram (TEG)***						
R value	4-8 min.				FFP (cryo, factor VIIa)	
K—value	0-4 min.				cryo (FFP, factor VIIa)	
α (angle)	47°-74°				cryo (FFP, factor VIIa)	
MA	54-72 mm				Platelets	

ECLS Anticoagulation QM Tool							Page 2
Date			Specialist			Patient	MR#
Protocol *	qam		prn	Hep, ACT, ATIII, Anti Xa, PT/PTT, fibrinogen, CBC, platelet, TEG			
	q12h		prn	ATIII, H/H, Platelet			
	q1h		prn	ACT			
*Record hourly levels and intervention							
Worksheet	Range	Time	Value	Intervention	Considerations		*Dose
Heparin (U/kg/hr)	25-50 U/Kg/hr	900			Higher flow lower ACT, lower flow higher ACT		**see protocol
ACT							
Heparin (U/kg/hr)	25-50 U/Kg/hr	1000					
ACT							
Heparin (U/kg/hr)	25-50 U/Kg/hr	1100					
ACT							
Heparin (U/kg/hr)	25-50 U/Kg/hr	1200					
ACT							
Heparin (U/kg/hr)	25-50 U/Kg/hr	1300					
ACT							
Heparin (U/kg/hr)	25-50 U/Kg/hr	1400					
ACT							
Heparin (U/kg/hr)	25-50 U/Kg/hr	1500					
ACT							
Heparin (U/kg/hr)	25-50 U/Kg/hr	1600			Higher flow lower ACT, lower flow higher ACT		**see protocol
ACT	160-180 sec.				Higher flow lower ACT, lower flow higher ACT		**see protocol
Heparin (U/kg/hr)	25-50 U/Kg/hr	1700					
ACT	160-180 sec.						
Heparin (U/kg/hr)	25-50 U/Kg/hr	1800					
ACT	160-180 sec.						
Heparin (U/kg/hr)	25-50 U/Kg/hr	1900					
ACT	160-180 sec.						

ECLS Anticoagulation QM Tool						Page 3	
Date			Specialist		Patient		
Protocol *	qam	prn	Hep, ACT, ATIII, Anti Xa, Pt/PTT, fibrinogen, platelet, TEG				
	q12h	prn	ATIII, H/H, Platelet				
	q1h	prn	ACT				
*Record hourly levels and intervention							
Worksheet	Range	Time	Value	Intervention	Considerations	*Dose	
Heparin (U/kg/hr)	25–50 U/Kg/hr	2000			Higher flow lower ACT, lower flow higher ACT	**see protocol	
ACT	160–180 sec.				Higher flow lower ACT, lower flow higher ACT	**see protocol	
H/H	Hct 35%–45%				VO$_2$, CO, SVR	10 mL/kg PRBCs	
AT III	60%–100%				Give FFP/ATIII if ACT low and heparin is high	FFP 20 mL/kg, ATIII	
Platelet Count	> 80,000				> 100,000 for bypass initiation then > 80,000	< 10 Kg - 10 mL/kg	
Heparin (U/kg/hr)	25–50 U/Kg/hr	2100					
ACT	160–180 sec.						
Heparin (U/kg/hr)	25–50 U/Kg/hr	2200					
ACT	160–180 sec.						
Heparin (U/kg/hr)	25–50 U/Kg/hr	2300					
ACT	160–180 sec.						
Heparin (U/kg/hr)	25–50 U/Kg/hr	2400			Higher flow lower ACT, lower flow higher ACT	**see protocol	
ACT	160–180 sec.				Higher flow lower ACT, lower flow higher ACT	**see protocol	
Heparin (U/kg/hr)	25–50 U/Kg/hr	01:00					
ACT	160–180 sec.						

Heparin (U/kg/hr)	25–50 U/Kg/hr	02:00				
ACT	160–180 sec.					
Heparin (U/kg/hr)	25–50 U/Kg/hr	03:00				
ACT	160–180 sec.					
Heparin (U/kg/hr)	25–50 U/Kg/hr	04:00			Higher flow lower ACT, lower flow higher ACT	**see protocol
ACT	160–180 sec.				Higher flow lower ACT, lower flow higher ACT	**see protocol
Heparin (U/kg/hr)	25–50 U/Kg/hr	05:00				
ACT	160–180 sec.					
Heparin (U/kg/hr)	25–50 U/Kg/hr	06:00				
ACT	160–180 sec.					
Heparin (U/kg/hr)	25–50 U/Kg/hr	07:00				
ACT	160–180 sec.					

ECLS Anticoagulation QM Tool			References	Page 4
** Heparin Protocol				Notes
ACT < 160	20 units heparin	repeat ACT 10 minutes		
repeat ACT < 160	20 units heparin	Increase heparin infusion by 10 U/kg, repeat ACT 10 minutes		Heparin 25-50 U/kg
repeat ACT < 160	20 units heparin	Increase heparin infusion by 5 U/kg, repeat ACT 10 minutes		Check ATIII level
repeat ACT < 160	20 units heparin	Increase heparin infusion by 5 U/kg, repeat ACT 10 minutes		FFP 10 mL/kg
repeat ACT < 160	call MD	Check heparin and anti Xa level		
ACT > 180		Decrease heparin by 5 U/kg		
ACT > 180		Decrease heparin by 5 U/kg		Heparin 25-50 U/kg
ACT > 180		Decrease heparin by 5 U/kg		Check ATIII, Plts, PT
ACT > 180	call MD	Check heparin and anti Xa level		Fibrinogen, heparin, Xa
*** DOSES Platelets				
< 10 kg		10mL/kg		Platelets < 80,000
> 10 kg		1 U/kg		Platelets < 80,000
Factor VII		90 mcg/kg q 2 hours		massive hemorrhage
Cryoprecipitate		1 unit per 5 kg		Fibrinogen < 100
Amicar		50 mg/kg bolus, 1-40 mg/kg/hr		FDP > 40
Argatroban		0.75 mcg/kg.min for 2 hours, inc. 0.1 mcg/kg/min until PTT 60		HIT
r-tPA		0.48 mg/kg bolus, 0.27 mg/kg/hr for 6 hours		life-threatening clot

FFP		1 mL/kg increases ATIII 1%		20 mL/kg
ATIII—Antithrombin III		**Recombinant Antithrombin III—(rATIII)**		
Thrombate		1 U increases ATIII 1% (1u/mL)		75 U/kg
ATRYN		1 U increases ATIII 1% (1u/mL)		75 U/kg
TEG***				
R = thrombin formation			FFP (cryo, factor VIIa)	4-8 min.
K = thrombin and fibrin formation			cryo (FFP, factor VIIa)	0-4 min.
α (angle)			cryo (FFP, factor VIIa)	47°-74°
MA = platelet function			platelets	54-72 mm

CHAPTER 8

Weaning and Idling for AV-ECMO for Infants

- As the patient's lungs improve, less ECMO flow will be needed to maintain the pO_2 70-80 mmHg and a mixed venous saturation > 70%.
- When the flow rate is 50% or less of the cardiac output, adjustments may need to be made.
- The ECMO physician may increase the FiO_2 to the ventilator.
- Ventilator adjustments will be made dependent upon the blood gas results.
- **Temperature regulation of the baby may change as the ECMO flow is decreased.** The overhead radiant warmer may need to have the temperature increased to maintain the baby's temperature as well as support heat exchange from the ECMO circuit.
- Often, lung improvement in the neonate is rapid. In a few hours, the flow rate can be decreased by as much as 50%.
- If the pO_2 is greater than 90 mmHg, the flow may be continuously turned down.
- The venous saturations should also be used as a guideline for weaning. Maintaining the saturations 70%-80%, with the saturations being in the upper range, usually indicate that the baby is ready to be weaned.
- Decrease the flow in relatively small increments (10-20 mL) and assess the status with the venous saturations and blood gases at frequent intervals.
- When the flow rate is at 30 mL/kg/min (resting cardiac output for a newborn is estimated at approximately 100 mL/min), then "idling" is achieved for an infant < = 3.5 kg baby.

- The baby will remain at this flow rate for four to eight hours to be sure that the improvement is not transient.
- In most babies, improvement continues while idling, and the ventilator settings may be decreased.

Open-Bridge ECMO / Idling

- Infants who are less than 3.5 kg may require an ECMO flow lower than 100 mL/min.
- Generally, a flow of 30%-40% of estimated resting cardiac output is appropriate for idle flow.
- A 2.5 kg infant may require or idle less than 75 mL/min flow (2.5 kg × 100 mL/min × 0.3 = 75 mL/min).
- Flows below 300 mL/min may decrease the ECMO flow to a rate below rated flow of the membrane.
- This may promote clot formation within the circuit if allowed for a period of time.
- This may decrease membrane function.
- When ECMO flow is expected to be less than 100 mL/min, then a partial-resistance clamp should be placed on the bridge (open bridge).
- Placing a partial-resistance clamp on the bridge will allow partial flow through the bridge.
- Titrated flow appropriate for the smaller infant will occur while diverting and maintaining the ECMO circuit flows at a higher rate.
    - reduce clot formation, membrane dysfunction
- The total ECMO circuit total flow should be maintained at 300 mL/min.
- When a partial-resistance clamp is placed on the bridge, flowmeters **must** be placed on the circuit to monitor patient and circuit flows separately.
- One flow probe must be placed on the arterial cannula, proximal to the patient, between the bridge and the patient.
- **Correct placement, orientation, and monitoring of the probes and flow are critical.**
- Directly measure the flow going to the patient.
- Adjust the amount of flow to the patient.
    - Maintain the pump flow at a constant 300 mL/min.
    - Adjust the partial-resistance clamp, slightly more open or closed, to achieve the desired flow to the patient as measured by the flow probe on the arterial catheter.

- This open-bridge idling may also be utilized for complex and marginal ECMO patients who have failed previous attempts to idle and wean or have been very unstable.
- When performing open bridge flow,

    o If the mixed venous saturation probe is placed after the bridge, the mixed venous saturation reading may increase due to recirculation in the circuit.

- The greater the amount of recirculation through the bridge, the higher the mixed venous saturation will record. This is not an accurate measurement of the patient-mixed venous saturation. Caution should be observed if the mixed venous saturation increases beyond 80%-85%, as this may be an indication of significant recirculation and inadequate patient flow. Check the patient flow probe. The pump will measure the total flow in the circuit.
- All blood gases to determine patient condition during open-bridge idling should be

    o Drawn from the patient or
    o Performed with the bridge **clamped** and the pump flow reduced to the total desired closed bridge idle flow for fifteen minutes.

    - Example for a 2.5 kg infant: the total closed bridge pump flow will be reduced to 75 mL/min as in the above reference
    - The bridge may then be opened after the blood gas and the partial-resistance clamp reinitiated at the desired flow for continued open-bridge idling with the pump flow increased back to 300 mL/min

- During idling, once improvement is determined not to be transient, it may be advantageous to change the endotracheal tube. It is easier to do this while on ECMO as the procedure can be done without concern about the time factor. It is, however, very important to remember that the baby is still heparinized and that every effort to avoid trauma should be made. The most experienced intubator should perform the procedure to ensure that a smooth intubation occurs. An airway exchange catheter may be used during reintubation to avoid excessive trauma.

- This open-bridge idling may also be utilized for complex and marginal ECMO patients who have failed previous attempts to idle and wean or have been very unstable.
- In the instance that rapid weaning is desired (i.e., bleeding or seizures), the ventilator settings may be adjusted more vigorously.
- Pulmonary function tests may also be performed while idling. These tests may give a better indication of the pulmonary function of the baby.
- The surgical team needs to be notified of the patient's condition and status of weaning and idling.

Weaning / Idling for VV-ECMO

- The infant's progress will show better arterial saturations.
- Venous saturations will stabilize and may increase as the arterial saturation increases.
- ABGs should be used to confirm the improvement.
- The ECMO pump flow may be gradually weaned by 10-20 mL increments until the effective flow reaches 40 mL/kg/min or minimum of 150 mL/min.
- The FiO_2 will usually need to be increased during this wean.
- Increase the ventilator to acceptable decannulation settings and repeat the ABG when the flow reaches 40 mL/kg/min or minimum of 150 mL/min.
- Repeat the ABG in fifteen minutes.
- If acceptable, repeat the ABG in one hour.
- Adjust ventilator as required. Idle may proceed for four to eight hours.
- The child who has achieved acceptable blood gases on lower VV-ECMO flows with the FiO_2 lowered to 0.5 is ready for a trial off.
- Trial-off VV-ECMO may be successfully performed by discontinuing the delivery of oxygen and all gas flow to the membrane while continuing the VV-ECMO flow with the bridge clamped.
- This will provide a good estimation of native lung function and oxygenation.

Trial Off / Decannulation

- After a successful weaning and idling period have been completed, the next step toward decannulation is a trial-off period.
- This is the period when

- o the cannulae are clamped;
- o the ECMO circuit recirculates through the patient bypass bridge; and
- o the baby is relying completely on the intrinsic cardiac, lung function, and ventilator support.

Once the ECMO physician orders the trial off, a few preparatory steps must be taken.

- All IV fluids infusing into the pump must be switched to a patient site and given time to stabilize.
- The heparin drip must be switched to a patient site at the same rate as before.
  - o Central line if available
  - o Purge line to start heparin at patient
- A nonheparinized port must be available for ACT sampling from the patient.
- The patient is now ready for trial off.
- The baby is taken trialed off as per bypass as per circuit protocol.
- The ECMO physician and a respiratory therapist are at the bedside to make necessary changes on the ventilator.

ECMO Specialist Responsibilities during Trial Off

- ACTs are performed every fifteen minutes on both the patient and pump.
- Heparin boluses may be given to both sites as needed.
- ACT range should be maintained 180-200.
- Flash the cannulas every fifteen minutes for approximately fifteen to thirty seconds.
  - o During cannula flash, do the following:
    1. Decrease extracorporeal flow rate
    2. Open arterial catheter
    3. Clamp bridge
    4. Open the venous catheter
    5. Wean ventilator settings as per ECMO physician
       a. Maintain a pO_2 of 70-100 torr
       b. Maintain pCO_2 35-45 torr
       c. Arterial saturations 90%-100%
       d. Perform ABGs as indicated to evaluate tolerance by the patient (vein-bridge-artery)

Weaning / Trial-Off Note

The ECMO pump flow is maintained at 200-300 mL/min. There must be a note in documenting the initiation of weaning and patient's tolerance during the procedure. Trial-off note should include the following:

- Who performed the procedure
- How it was performed
- Patient condition
- Procedures
- IV fluid placement
- Medications
- ACT management
- Completed trial-off checklist

Decannulation

The ECLS *trial-off* sequence can affect coagulation and oxygenation status. It is the purpose important to standardize the trial off. Once a patient is *clamped off* from the extracorporeal circuit, the clinical condition and manipulation of the patient can all negatively affect the outcome of the trial off.

Monitoring and controlling cardiac output, blood pressure, oxygenation, and ventilation affect the outcome of the trial off.

4. With a physician present, adjust ventilation and pharmacological hemodynamic support to *off ECLS* settings.
5. Arterial saturation by pulse oximeter and SvO_2 should both rise as a response to these adjustments.
6. Move all medications to a peripheral venous line of the patient (when possible) or to the arterial line.
    a. Note any drug incompatibilities from combining separate intravenous infusions that were isolated by the ECLS circuit.
7. With the ECFR is at idle (100 mL/minute), note the exact time and clamp off the patient.
8. Clamp the venous line (patient side of the bridge), remove the clamp on the bridge, clamp the arterial line (patient side of the bridge) (vein-bridge-artery).
9. Increase the flow in the circuit to 300 mL/min (unless contraindicated).
10. Turn the gas sweep to zero.

11. Confirm by SvO$_2$ monitor that the circuit saturation is greater than 98% sat. If not, turn the sweep to 1 lpm for two minutes then turn off.
12. At approximately ten minutes after the trial has begun, draw and analyze the circuit ACT.
13. At approximately fifteen minutes after the trial has begun, do as follows:

    a. Draw the following blood, in order, from the patient's arterial line
    b. Draw the arterial blood gas into the preheparinized syringe (5 mL of arterial blood, or as much up to five that the patient can tolerate)
    c. Draw 0.1 mL in a **nonheparinized** syringe for the patient ACT

14. Decrease the extracorporeal flow rate to 100 mL.
15. Open the circuit to the patient by performing the following:

    a. For occlusion pump circuits, open the clamp on the arterial line (patient side of the bridge), place the clamp on the patient bridge, open the clamp on the venous line (artery-bridge-vein).
    b. For centrifugal pump circuits, open the venous clamp, place on the bridge, open the arterial clamp.

16. Increase the flow to 200 mL/minute for two minutes (unless contraindicated).

    a. Two minutes will mix the patient circuit blood volume by 100%. The circuit does not metabolize heparin, so the ACT of the patient should be within 10% of the circuit. If not, adequate mixing of patient and circuit blood did not occur.

17. Watch the SvO$_2$ carefully. Note the **lowest** value that is attained once the patient is back on ECLS. The lowest value is the **patient's SvO$_2$ off ECMO**.
18. If the value falls below 70%, assess the patient for either ventilatory or hemodynamic stability. (Did the blood pressure drop? How was the blood gas?)
19. Discuss this data with the ECMO physician and make the appropriate adjustments.

20. Next time on bypass, reassess that initial SvO_2 for improvement secondary to the changes that were made.
21. Decrease the flow to 100 mL/minute.
22. Clamp off the patient. Clamping the venous line (patient side of the bridge), remove the clamp on the bridge, clamp the arterial line (patient side of the bridge) (vein-bridge-artery).
23. Restart the fifteen-minute clock and repeat the above steps.
24. Once stable, ascertain that the circuit SvO_2 returns to 98% or above. If not, oxygenate the blood with 1 lpm for thirty seconds. Note: if blood gases are unavailable on a fifteen-minute basis, rely on patient oximeter saturations, blood pressures, and the "lowest sat" when flashing the circuit.
25. The trial-off period is approximately one hour.
26. If the baby is tolerating and the decision to decannulate is made, the baby is placed back on bypass (at 200 mL/min for newborn) while waiting for the surgical team to arrive.
27. Decannulation occurs in the same manner as the cannulation procedure.
28. Sterile technique is closely adhered to.
29. Don proper personal protection equipment (PPE), including surgical hat, mask, and gloves as when assembling sterile equipment and tubing pack.
30. The same personnel are at the bedside (except for the perfusionist).

ECMO specialist duties during decannulation:

- Remove the patient from bypass as per protocol when the surgical team is present.
- Continue to perform ACTs every fifteen minutes until the incision is opened. You may discontinue the heparin drip at this time.
- The ECMO pump may be turned off when the cannulae are removed.
- All ECMO equipment must be thoroughly cleaned as per protocol.
- The cart must be restocked, and everything must be returned to the ECMO storeroom. Approximately one to one-and-a-half hours after decannulation, an ACT should be performed from a patient nonheparinized port.

Documentation during decannulation:

1. Vital signs q15" (HR, B/P, CVP, SaO_2) until one hour postdecannulation.

2. Clean area observed and surgical attire in use.
3. Personnel involved with procedure.
4. Time of paralyzation, if not already paralyzed.
5. Time of IV fluids switched to patient.
6. Time of decannulation, bypass terminated.
7. Ventilator changes.
8. Patient's tolerance to the procedure.
9. If a graft was used for cannulation (ask cannulating surgeon), continue heparin and ACTs for approximately one hour after the cannulae was removed.
10. Decannulation note.

    a. This note should include the following:
        i. Time-out protocol
        ii. Decannulation checklist
        iii. Time begun
        iv. Surgeons / physicians present
        v. Sterile technique observed
        vi. Patient condition
        vii. Medications given
        viii. Procedures
        ix. Complications
        x. Time finished

Stinting

The patient on extracorporeal life support may require an immediate removal from the circuit (clotting-embolus) or is clinically questionable as to whether the patient can continue to tolerate the removal of ECLS. It is for these reasons that "stinting" or removing the ECLS circuit, leaving the ECLS cannulae in the neck, is used as another weaning tool. By keeping the cannulae in for 24 degrees, returning to ECLS is simplified, removing the surgical cannulation procedure from the time that the patient qualifies for ECLS to the actual time that life support is restarted.

Physician, perfusionist, or the extracorporeal specialist may only perform this procedure.

1. Establish the necessity for stinting and verify that the attending is aware of the necessity for the procedure.
2. Assemble the following shopping list:

a. Two sterile ¼" × male Luer connectors
   b. Sterile Betadine swabs
   c. Four tubing clamps
   d. Sterile scalpel blade
   e. Two sterile stopcocks
   f. Two IV sets with two units per mL heparin in normal saline
   g. Sterile gloves (in package)
   Two twenty mL syringes with two units heparin per mL saline

3. Move all infusions from the ECLS circuit to the patient. (If vascular access is minimal, the jugular ECLS catheter can be used for infusions.)
4. Clinically monitor the patient to determine if the patient has tolerated the trial-off protocol
5. Send appropriate blodd gas, chest xray and labs
6. Verify that ventilator settings are appropriate and remove the patient from ECLS (vein-bridge-artery).
7. If the patient does not tolerate the trial-off protocol, notify ECMO physician.
8. Sterile technique is closely adhered to.
9. Don proper personal protection equipment (PPE), including surgical hat, mask, and gloves as when assembling sterile equipment and tubing pack.
10. Create sterile work area under cannula.
11. Open the sterile gloves near the cannulas, leaving the paper as a part of the sterile work field.
12. Have the bedside nurse open the ¼" × male Luer connectors, Betadine swabs, sterile scalpel blade, and the sterile scalpel blade onto the field.
13. Starting with the venous side, swab the area with Betadine approximately 3 cm from the distal end of the ECLS catheters. (The venous will be easier secondary to the patient's arterial versus venous hemodynamic pressures.)
14. Squeezing the Betadine tubing between your fingers until the blood in the squeezed tubing is displaced (tubing clear), clamp both sides of the cleaned tubing with tubing clamps.
15. Fold the tubing between clamps until a crease is seen.
16. Lay the scalpel blade gently onto the crimped tubing, cutting the tubing.
17. Insert the ¼" × Luer connector into the tubing attached to the catheter.
18. Attach the stopcock to the male Luer.

19. Attach the 20 mL syringe of heparinized saline to the stopcock.
20. Open the stopcock to the catheter and exert a light negative pressure on the syringe, sucking any air bubbles into the top of the syringe, and carefully open the tubing clamp; air and blood should enter the syringe.
21. Once the air has been removed, slowly infuse the heparinized saline into the catheter until flushed clean.
22. Turn the stopcock off to the patient, attach the IV infusion, and start the IV rate at 2 mL/hr.
23. Repeat steps 8 through 17 on the arterial catheter.
24. Stabilize catheters to bed, as if the patient is on ECLS.
25. If the patient is stable, with orders from the physician, at this time, the ECLS specialist may turn off the pump, heater, and gas sweep.

Chapter 9

Emergencies

Mechanical Circulatory Support

Perioperative Cardiac Surgery

Perioperative cardiac support is the most common application of ECLS in the world.[22] Surgery for congenital heart disease with severe low cardiac output state may be refractory to maximal medical management. Mechanical circulatory support may allow salvage of many of these challenging patients. The field of pediatric mechanical circulatory support is evolving rapidly.

Two forms of mechanical support are currently available to infants and children:

- The ventricular assist device (VAD)
- Extracorporeal membrane oxygenation (ECMO)

Each technique has advantages and disadvantages.

The intra-aortic balloon pump is a balloon catheter that is placed into the descending aorta usually through the femoral artery. This balloon then inflates during diastole to provide hemodynamic augmentation. The IABP also increases diastolic coronary blood flow and decreases left ventricular afterload. It is rarely applied to infants and children.

Unfortunately, the IABP has numerous disadvantages in the pediatric population. Hemodynamic augmentation is often inadequate because of the compliant elastic aortic wall in children. Vascular problems occur with insertion because of the small femoral artery size. The rapid heart rate in many children interferes with timing of the intra-aortic balloon. Finally, the balloon has been reported to occasionally occlude the superior mesenteric artery and renal artery as well as cause severe limb ischemia.

Three types of **ventricular assist device** may be utilized:

- The left ventricular assist device (LVAD)

    o The LVAD will assist left ventricular function by pumping blood from the left atrium to the aorta. This device has been shown to be extremely useful in adults with ischemic heart disease and isolated left ventricular dysfunction. Children with left ventricular dysfunction are less likely to have preserved right ventricular function and pulmonary function. Nevertheless, in cases of isolated left ventricular dysfunction, the LVAD has been utilized with eventual survival of 40%-70%.

- The right ventricular assist device (RVAD)

    o Isolated right ventricular dysfunction can be treated with a RVAD, which will pump blood from the right atrium to the pulmonary artery. Cases of isolated right ventricular dysfunction are uncommon in the pediatric population.

- The biventricular assist device (BiVAD)

    o A BiVAD can be utilized in cases of biventricular dysfunction. This form of support utilizes both an LVAD and an RVAD. Biventricular dysfunction without pulmonary dysfunction is rare in children. Furthermore, BiVAD utilization can be technically challenging in smaller children.

- Advantages of ventricular assist devices include providing good oxygen delivery to the tissues as well as unloading the supported ventricle to allow time for ventricular healing. Also, the VAD will allow for lower levels of anticoagulation then ECMO.
- Disadvantages of VAD include bleeding complications, potential pulmonary dysfunction necessitating conversion to ECMO, potential renal dysfunction necessitating hemofiltration, and potential for infection.

Extracorporeal Membrane Oxygenation

- ECMO utilizes venoarterial bypass with a membrane oxygenator. This technique allows both hemodynamic and pulmonary support. ECMO has been utilized with increased frequency to provide postcardiotomy support for children with severe cardiopulmonary dysfunction with pulmonary dysfunction after surgery for congenital heart disease. Survival in many centers now exceeds 50%.
- Advantages of ECMO include the possibility of providing total cardiopulmonary support and allowing for cardiac and pulmonary healing. Although this may be accomplished with venous drainage from the right atrium and inflow into the aorta, many centers feel it is important to decompress the left side of the heart as well with an additional drainage catheter in the left atrium.
- Disadvantages of ECMO include the need for higher levels of anticoagulation compared to other forms of support. This anticoagulation leads to the additional disadvantages of bleeding, blood product requirements, multiple reexplorations to control hemorrhage, and potential for infection.
- Future research in mechanical cardiopulmonary support for children centers on decreasing requirements for anticoagulation and thus decreasing bleeding and infectious complications. Coated circuits are being studied in multiple centers, which seem to offer numerous advantages and disadvantages. Further research should lead to more biocompatible support systems as well as smaller support systems. The eventual possibility of developing implantable support systems for long-term system in children is appealing but logistically challenging.

Patient Emergencies

An understanding of the physiology relevant to ECMO, familiarity with the ECMO circuit and with basic circuit procedures, and the attainment of a certain level of confidence in managing patients on ECMO prepare one to handle most of the problems routinely encountered with this technique. However, potentially catastrophic complications arise unexpectedly and progress rapidly.

Sudden Cardiorespiratory Decompensation during ECMO

- Major cardiac dysfunction is usually not appreciated during VA bypass given that at least 120 mL/min/kg flow can be provided. Because some

degree of cardiac depression is fairly common early in the course of ECMO runs, particularly with the more severely asphyxiated infants, VA bypass is warranted over VV bypass in these cases.
- If an infant suffers a cardiac arrest, develops a malignant dysrrhythmia, or drops his cardiac output secondary to severe myocardial dysfunction, the treatment of choice while on ECMO is simply to turn up the pump flow. This may require the addition of blood volume to the circuit. The cause of the acute event can then be determined and treated. Continued ECMO support is likely to be one of the most effective therapeutic measures. Treatment may include the administration of standard "arrest" medications, some adjustments of the electrolyte levels, the addition of an antiarrhythmic agent, treatment with sympathomimetics or inotropes, or even countershock therapy.
- If the pump flow cannot be increased sufficiently to compensate for the fall in intrinsic cardiac output, then the episode must be handled much the same as cardiac arrest in any other patient. The most common cause of cardiac dysfunction in ventilated neonates is of **respiratory**, not *cardiac failure*. First, check the endotracheal tube, listen for breath sounds, and hand ventilate the baby, noting the PIP at all times. Think about inadvertent extubation or the development of a tension pneumothorax. Remember that the reason you cannot achieve the desired ECMO flows may be that venous return to the patient's heart is being impeded because of an accumulation of blood or air in the chest or pericardium. Assign someone to begin chest compressions, bearing in mind that the infant is still heparinized, and administer the routine cardiotropic drugs. In the event of acute cardiac decompensation, assure that a malfunction of the ECMO system is not the cause.
- Extreme acid-base imbalance caused by the addition of too much or too little carbon dioxide to the sweep gas, hypoxia caused by the tubing to the gas inlet port of the oxygenator disconnecting, or hypovolemia from failure to clamp the main bridge are examples of the ways in which circuit problems can precipitate such an event.

CPS and Cardiac Support for Emergencies

1. Support for cardiac diagnosis

Support for patients with a primary cardiac diagnosis is preferably provided by the cardiopulmonary support (CPS) system in the cardiac intensive care unit. The assisted venous drainage of the CPS circuit allows for optimal cardiac support without need for additional vents or cannulae. In addition, the coating of a circuit reduces thrombosis and bleeding. Preoperative and postoperative support as well as CPS best provides support for acute cardiomyopathy. For those protocols, refer to the CPS policy and protocol manual.

2. CPS and ECMO

The CPS system and ECMO system complement each other in several ways. Each case is considered on an individual basis.

3. Rescue CPS

The low crystalloid priming volume and the rapid deployment capability of the CPS circuit make it ideal when support must be initiated emergently. An unstable patient may benefit from emergent CPS support: ninety seconds to prime plus cannulation. There is an emergency cannulation tray in the operating room that allows cannulation with minimal OR support if necessary. The downside of emergent CPS support followed by transition to ECMO is, of course, exposure to two circuits in a short period of time.

4. ECMO to CPS

The CPS circuit is coated in its entirety. Patients with correctable bleeding issues may benefit from a short period of CPS support without heparinization while these bleeding issues are corrected (usually surgically). The downside is again the exposure to an additional circuit.

The portability and transportability of the CPS circuit make it suitable for transfer of patients already on ECMO at another institution. Transport is optimally performed in an airworthy aircraft; the airworthiness certification of the portable CPS circuit only applies to that aircraft.

5. CPS to ECMO

Patients on the CPS circuit with resolution of cardiac issues but with remaining medical support issues (usually pulmonary and/or infectious) may benefit from transition to the ECMO circuit for longer-term support.

Emergency Decannulation

In the event the patient's condition requires an emergency termination of ECMO support, the ECMO physician will initiate the termination of bypass using the following general guidelines:

- The surgical team must be notified about the patients' condition immediately.
- The ECMO specialist will wean the flow down to idle speed.

- o The rate at which weaning occurs should be over two to three hours, dependent on what flow the weaning process was started or why the wean is being done.
- o Flow may be weaned 50-100 mL per hour for neonates and 100-300 mL per hour for pediatric patients.

- Ventilator settings are increased to support the patient when the flow is approximately 50% of cardiac output or when the venous saturations are compromised.
- Inotropic support may be instituted at any time as per physician discretion.
- The trial-off procedure should be initiated just prior to the surgical procedure.
- ACTs should be maintained 180-200 seconds until the cannulae are removed.
- All patients will follow the decannulation procedure scheduled. This includes those patients who have a "do not resuscitate" (DNR) order.

Differential Diagnosis of Acute Decompensation

Pericardial Tamponade (Due to Air or Blood)

- HR up then down, BP down, pulse pressure narrowed, CVP increased, marked rise in paO_2, followed by fall in ECMO flow and poor perfusion.
- Management includes decompressing the pericardium acutely then surgical placement of pericardial drain. Control bleeding, CXR, echo.

Tension Hemo/Pneumothorax

- Chest distended, not moving well with ventilated breaths. First a fall then a marked rise in paO_2 followed by BP down, pulse down, ECMO flow down, and poor perfusion.
- Management includes decompressing the chest acutely then surgical placement of chest tube (with cautery). Control bleeding, transilluminate, CXR.

Respiratory Failure

- Endotracheal tube "out," ventilator malfunction.
- Management includes check ETT, ventilator, ECMO circuit.

Electrolyte Imbalance, Myocardial Ischemia, Drug Effects, Infection

- Dysrrhythmia, HR up or down, BP down, poor perfusion, poor contractility on echo.
- Management includes support cardiac output with ECMO, drugs, fluid, CXR, EKG, echo. Oxygenate, correct electrolytes, treat infection.

Massive Hemorrhage (Especially Intracranial)

- Pallor or cyanosis, HR up then down, HCT down, BP down, perfusion poor. In the newborn, may see a sudden rash or change in the color of the upper chest, neck, or head or no clinical change if on ECMO.
- Management includes brain ultrasound, CXR. Aspirate stomach, stool blood test, abdominal ultrasound. Maintain ACTs 160-180, platelet count 100,000 or greater. Consider Amicar (see Amicar).

Overwhelming Sepsis

- Shock, poor perfusion, DIC.
- Management includes sepsis workup (no spinal tap). Change antibiotics, vasopressors, volume, correct DIC, etc.

Abnormal Bleeding

- Bleeding is not rare during ECMO. Some oozing from the cannula incision is fairly common. However, serious bleeding is not routine and must be addressed aggressively.
- Coagulopathy is related to Virchow's factors of coagulation: flow, circulating factors, and endothelium.
- Low flow ECMO potentiates the low flow characteristics that promote coagulopathies.
- Increasing the ECMO flow will ameliorate these factors and lead to a reduced requirement for anticoagulation and reduced clotting.
- Reduced clotting will increase circulating cofactors (consumption coagulopathy) and reduce hemorrhage.
- If hemorrhage is life threatening or surgery is unsuccessful, contraindicated, or worsening bleeding, then the heparin may be turned off with high ECMO flow rates.
- Consider HIT.
- The highest flow allowed by the patient is preferred.

- A new circuit may be primed at the bedside and immediately available.
- Amicar should be turned off, preferably thirty minutes prior.
- Constant inspection of the circuit for clots is required.

Intracranial Hemorrhage

Daily head ultrasounds should be obtained to evaluate the patient for an ICH. Once a grade I or II or other intracerebral hemorrhage is diagnosed, management of such bleeds includes maintaining the platelet count 150,000 or greater and managing ACTs 160-180 seconds. These precautions will help limit the bleed from extending.

If the IVH or ICH extends, the decision to discontinue ECMO therapy and return to conventional treatment will be evaluated.

If a grade III or greater is diagnosed initially, the decision must be made to discontinue ECMO therapy and return to conventional treatment.

Cannula Site Hemorrhage

Some slight initial oozing is expected from the cannula site(s). However, if the oozing becomes serious, requiring frequent dressing changes and replacement volume, more aggressive measures need to be taken.

The use of Gelfoam with thrombin and calcium topically has proven to be effective in some cases. The Gelfoam is cut to size (to cover the area bleeding the most) and saturated with thrombin (mixed as per manufacturer's recommendations). Using sterile technique, this is applied with direct pressure for five minutes to the area of bleeding. The site is then dressed with sterile four by fours and plastic tape. Should the dressing require changing, the Gelfoam/thrombin piece is not to be removed. This may dislodge any clot formation that may have occluded.

Fibrin glue. Occasionally, in extreme cases of bleeding, the Gelfoam/thrombin mixture may not be adequate. Another intervention recommended is the use of fibrin glue sealant. A combination of **crossmatched cryoprecipitate, thrombin, and CaCl** is applied to the site. Within seconds, a clot is formed. The fibrin sealant forms a bond that interlocks with the molecular structure of the damaged tissue and begins mimicking the body's normal clotting mechanism. With the use of this mixture, hemostasis is achieved rapidly and safely.

Fibrin Glue Sealant Preparation and Application

- Separate 12 mL syringes.
- Draw 10 mL of cryoprecipitate in one syringe (crossmatched with the patient)
- CaCl 250 mg (2.5 mL) plus thrombin 7.5 mL (mixed as per manufacturer's policy) into the other syringe.
- Simultaneous injecting this solution onto the site with thorough mixing is achieved. This simultaneous mixing is preferred to sequential application because it achieves the greatest tensile strength and resultant immediate hemostasis.
- Once the mixture has been applied, the site should be dressed with sterile four by fours and plastic tape. When the dressing is changed, care should be taken not to dislodge the clot. This will interrupt any clotting that may have already taken effect.
- If the bleeding is extreme and will not be controlled by the recommended steps, reexploration of the site may be necessary by the surgeon.

Invasive Site Hemorrhage

Bleeding into the site of a previous invasive procedure happens often enough that it is necessary to monitor these locations in particular. Previous surgery, for example, to repair a congenital diaphragmatic hernia is a risk factor. Care must also be taken in assessing central line sites as these may start bleeding when ECMO is begun.

If the hemorrhage continues despite maintaining the platelet count greater than 150,000 and the ACTs 160-180 seconds, exploratory surgery may need to be considered.

Other Systems

Gastrointestinal bleeding has also been observed in the ECMO patient.
- Care must be taken to prevent bleeding.

    o NG tubes at low intermittent suction
    o Gastric protective medication administration
    o Maintaining ACTs between 160-180 seconds
    o Platelet count is greater than 100,000

- A GI bleed that is present may respond to the above measures plus iced saline lavage and medications. In extreme cases, vasopressin may be used.

- Esophageal bleeding may also occur even if precautions are taken. The same steps to treat this bleeding are taken; as for other bleeds, prevent if possible. Also, balloon tamponade may be necessary in extreme cases.

Air Emboli

- It is possible for a large bolus of air to develop and circulate rapidly into the infant. This complication, although rare, is commonly fatal.
- There are several potential sources of such an emboli.
- paO2 in the blood is very high (> 400 torr), oxygen can very easily be forced out of solution.
- Hitting the membrane or operating system in a low ambient pressure environment (such as in flight in a nonpressurized cabin) may produce veritable foam in the top of the oxygenator
- Operating the pump with a clamp on the venous side of the circuit or with the pump controller in the override position may cause cavitation of a pressurized circuit
- Kinking the outlet arm of the bladder (as can occur during "walking" of the raceway) can generate a markedly negative pressure in the blood path and similarly pull large amounts of gas out of solution. The bladder box is designed to limit the occurrence of this problem.
- The most dramatic air embolus occurs when a small tear develops in the membrane, allowing blood to leak into the gas path of the oxygenator.
    - o The blood gradually moves down to the gas exhalation port where it may either be blown out in small drops or accumulate and form a clot.
    - o This clot obstructs the gas outlet; a large bolus of air will gush across the tear in the membrane into the blood path.
    - o The gas-trapping capacity of the device may rapidly be exceeded, and the embolus will push into the infant's aorta.
- Obviously, the ideal solution to this problem rests on prevention and rapid response.
    - o Keep the pO_2 in the postmembrane at 400 torr or less.
    - o Careful monitoring of the toggle switches on the pump controller.

- o Careful monitoring of the placement of extraneous clamps on the circuit.
- o Adherence to the precautions with regard to "walking" the raceway will eliminate the most common problems.
- o Touching the gas outlet port with your fingers as part of your hourly checks will alert the specialist that there is blood rather than water being expelled.
- o A combination of strict adherence to the hourly protocol and general vigilance for problems will permit the fastest-possible response time once an air embolus is detected.

- If a bolus of air is sighted but has not yet entered the patient, the techniques taught in the emergency process should be followed.

- o If the air is headed toward the arterial cannula, the pump should be turned off and a clamp placed on the arterial and venous cannulas closest to the baby. Ventilator settings should be set to emergency settings, and the physician should be notified. The air should then be removed as per emergency protocol.
- o If, however, air has already entered the patient, additional protective measures should be taken. Once the baby is off bypass, lower his head relative to his body as much as possible. Place in a left-side-down position. This may help to move any air pockets away from his cerebral circulation. Once the air has been removed from the circuit, the specialist then must determine the etiology of the problem.

Patent Ductus Arteriosus

- A PDA may be suspected in any infant. It is not necessarily limited to premature babies.
- A systolic murmur may not always be large. When listening for a murmur, remember that a continuous murmur with systolic augmentation is created by the jet effect at the arterial catheter.
- Symptoms include persistently poor perfusion, acidosis, edematous lungs, and low urine output.
- The ability to achieve extraordinarily high ECMO flow rates.

- o (i.e., over 500 mL in a 3-kg baby) without hypervolemia
- o The pulse pressure may remain wide even with increased ECMO flow rates.

- The clinical diagnosis may be confirmed using Doppler echocardiography or angiography.
- Surgical ligation may be safely performed during bypass.

    o   Special measures include maintaining the ACTs 160-1,800.
    o   Liberal use of electrocautery during surgery.
    o   Maximization of ECMO flow.
    o   Ongoing blood and volume replacement both during and after the case.

Chapter 10

Mechanical Emergencies on ECMO

Circuit Emergencies

Taking a Patient Off Pump for an Emergency

1. Shut off the pump (use the speed control knob).
2. Clamp arterial and venous lines above the bridge.
3. Open the patient bridge.
4. Turn off the sweep gas.
5. Have the ECMO physician called stat.
6. Institute the emergency ventilator settings (by RN or RRT).
7. Put circuit IV to patient if anticipating being off greater than fifteen minutes.
8. Evaluate the emergency and make a plan.
9. Turn the pump on and recirculate through the patient bridge if possible.
10. Fix the problem.
11. If patient is taken off bypass for more than three minutes or if physiologic changes occur earlier, when off bypass, all medications should be switched directly to the patient.

Changing the Oxygenator (Medtronic)

Supplies

- ER kit
- Oxygenator

- Cardiotomy reservoir and holder
- Two (2) ¼" tubing packages (10' length)
- Two (2) ¼ × ¼ connectors
- Two (2) pigtails
- Backup pump
- Two (2) 500 mL bags Plasmalyte-A
- IV spike
- CO_2 tank
- One (1) unit PRBCs
- Two hundred fifty (250) units heparin

Priming New Oxygenator (Medtronic)

- Place cardiotomy upside down in holder; remove 3/8" cap.
- Place oxygenator in the bracket; connect pigtails.
- Attach vacuum to gas outlet (leave off).
- Place O_2 filter and small piece of tubing on CO_2 tank and connect to gas inlet; turn on CO_2 for five minutes.
- Place ¼ tubing on oxygenator inlet through pump head to the bottom of the cardiotomy.
- Place ¼" tubing from oxygenator outlet to the top of the cardiotomy.
- Clamp oxygenator inlet and outlet lines after CO_2 flush is turned off, and turn on vacuum for three minutes.
- Prime cardiotomy reservoir with small piece of ¼ tubing and IV spike.
- Remove clamp from blood inlet line and rapid prime oxygenator.
- Remove clamp from oxygenator outlet line.
- Recirculate and debubble oxygenator.

*Oxygenator may be left primed like this for twenty-four hours if top Luer of cardiotomy is recapped.

Blood Priming New Oxygenator

- Remove oxygenator outlet line from top of cardiotomy.
- Turn on pump and drain prime from cardiotomy into basin.
- When cardiotomy is almost empty (10-15 mL left), add 1 unit PRBCs preheparinized with 250 units heparin.
- Turn on pump to prime oxygenator while draining prime out into basin.
- Turn off pump when blood prime is complete.

- Double clamp oxygenator inlet and outlet lines 2" from oxygenator.
- Cut tubing and attach connectors to each end.
- Cover ends with sterile caps from tubing.

Placing New Oxygenator in Line

- Double clamp oxygenator bridge 1" from each Y connector.
- Swab and cut tubing.
- Make airless connections with connectors on new oxygenator.
- Open clamps to new oxygenator and clamp inlet and outlet of old oxygenator.
- Recirculate to remove any air and go back on bypass as per protocol.
- Cut out old oxygenator and replace with new bridge.
- Come off bypass to recirculate through new bridge to remove any air.
- Go on bypass as per protocol.
- A second oxygenator can be safely placed "in parallel to the first, if physiologically indicated."

Priming New Heat Exchanger

- Heat exchanger
- Cardiotomy reservoir
- Two (2) ¼ tubing (10' length)
- Two (2) ¼ × ¼ connectors
- One (1) 1,000 mL bag Plasmalyte-A
- One (1) unit PRBCs (quadpacked)
- ER kit
- IV spike
- Backup pump
- One hundred (100) units heparin

Setup

- Place heat exchanger in bracket and cardiotomy upside own in holder; remove 3/8" cap.
- Connect water lines and water test.
- Connect ¼ tubing from blood inlet to bottom of cardiotomy.
- Connect ¼ tubing from blood outlet to top of cardiotomy.
- Prime oxygenator with a small piece of ¼ tubing and IV spike.
- Place tubing in pump head; set a gross occlusion and recirculate.

Blood Prime

- Remove blood outlet line from top of cardiotomy reservoir.
- Turn on pump and pump out prime into basin until reservoir is almost empty (10-15 mL).
- Add 1 split PRBCs preheparinized with 100 units heparin.
- Turn on pump and prime with blood while running out prime into basin.
- Double clamp 2" from inlet and outlet, swab with Betadine, and cut tubing.
- Add ¼ × ¼ connectors and cap with sterile caps.

Replace Heat Exchanger

- Come off bypass as per protocol.
- Double clamp 2" proximal and distal to ¼ connector.
- Remove ¼ connector.
- Connect tubing to connectors on new heat exchanger, making an airless connection.
- Remove clamps and recirculate.
- Go on bypass as per protocol.
- Reconnect water lines.

Chapter 11

Plasmapheresis

Introduction

Huang Di, the Yellow Emperor of China who reigned in the middle of the third millennium BCE, first introduced the concept of balancing circulating "forces" within the body to promote health and treat disease.[1] Galen popularized the concept of forces within the body, the "four humours," in the Roman Empire. Managing circulating humours was done routinely in an attempt to improve or restore health.[11] The Greek verb *aphaeresis*, meaning "to take away, withdraw, or separate," continues to be a central concept and application in Western medicine. The term *plasmapheresis* is used interchangeably for a variety of clinical applications. It may refer to the removal, exchange, modification, or filtration of circulating blood components, with or without the returning of a blood component. Therapeutic plasma exchange (TPE) is the most frequent plasma "pheresis" modality performed. TPE utilizes either a centrifuge or filter to separate or remove the plasma components and replace a plasma component concurrently. The goal is to remove, replace, or deplete unique circulating substances that are responsible for the disease process.

The process of removing cellular components (cytapheresis) includes red cell pheresis or erythrocytapheresis, which is the removal of red blood cells (PRBCs). Therapeutic leukodepletion is employed for the removal of large numbers of circulating white blood cells (WBCs) or granulocytes or monocytes, thereby decreasing aggregates that interfere with blood flow during the acute presentation of leukemia. Leukopheresis often refers to peripheral stem cell collection, which is performed to remove specific $CD_{34}+$ progenitor monocytes (WBCs) from peripheral blood for storage and reinfusion during the process of bone marrow transplantation.

The application of TPE includes infection, inflammatory, autoimmune, oncological, metabolic, neurological or renal diseases.[42] In the past ten years, many hospitals have developed apheresis programs due to the growing success and increased therapeutic use of this procedure.[43, 44] The technique has also gained widespread acceptance in Europe.[45] TPE is generally a supportive therapy used in conjunction with ongoing care and has been shown to increase the chance of recovery and survival in critically ill children and adults.[45-59]

Common Indications

Goodpasture's disease	Guillain-Barré
Acute inflammatory polyradiculoneuropathy	Acute inflammatory CNS demyelination
Kawasaki syndrome	Toxic shock
Meningococcemia	Purpura fulminans
Peritransplant incompatibilities	Systemic lupus erythematosus
Rheumatoid arthritis	Multiple sclerosis
Toxicologic emergencies	Hepatic coagulopathy
Myasthenia gravis	Stevens-Johnson syndrome
Polyneuropathy	Fulminant vasculitis
Thrombotic thrombocytopenic purpura	Hemolytic uremic syndrome
Heparin-induced thrombocytopenia	Hydrops
Idiopathic thrombotic diseases	Sepsis

Principles of TPE Operation

TPE, for the patient on ECMO, is performed in the intensive care unit by individuals who are ECMO certified or under the direct supervision of an ECMO specialist. The direct supervision of a qualified ECMO physician is also necessary. The patient's weight, sex, height, hematocrit, and procedure specific information are programmed into the machine software, and the machine is wheeled next to the ECMO circuit. A unique TPE circuit is loaded into a centrifugal machine for each therapy. The appropriate prescribed fluids are connected to the TPE, and the specific software program chosen for each therapy primes the circuit automatically. A filtration system may alternatively be used. Replacement fluids, anticoagulant, and priming solutions are dependent on size of patient and chosen before the therapy based on the child's condition.

The access to systemic circulation is drawn directly from the ECMO circuit without interruption or alteration of the ECMO flow. Once the TPE circuit is connected to the ECMO, circuit blood is pumped into the machine with an anticoagulant that is automatically calculated and added as the blood enters the centrifuge. A fully heparinized ECMO circuit may negate the need for additional anticoagulation. Heparinized or otherwise coated, ECMO circuits may affect the anticoagulation necessary for the TPE circuit. The need for additional or alternative anticoagulation should be evaluated for each patient and each therapy.

The centrifuge separates the blood into layers primarily based on molecular weight and density. Red cells are the densest and collect against the centrifuge wall first or farthest outside on the centrifuge plate, followed by white cells, platelets, and plasma. Centrifugal TPE utilizes optical sensors to detect each layer interface to minimize contamination of each cell and fluid layer. The desired components are automatically removed to collection bags, and the remaining blood components along with appropriate replacement fluids are returned to the patient. Rotary peristaltic pumps automatically control the amount of blood pumped from the patient, the amount of the component sent to the collection bag, the specific amount of anticoagulant, and when programmed, the appropriate constitution-reinfused fluids. Warmers can be added to the circuit to warm replacement fluid to prevent hypothermia caused by infusion of room temperature or cold fluids. This is generally unnecessary with a functioning heat exchanger during ECMO as these fluids are entered preheat exchanger. Most apheresis machines also have the capability of selecting the percentage of fluids for automatic reinfusion. This is done in direct proportion to the percentage of fluid removed, thus decreasing the possibility of the patient developing hypovolemia or hypervolemia. Multiple audiovisual alarms alert the operator to potential problems.

TPE may also be performed using a filtration technique. An anticoagulated extracorporeal circuit passes the blood through a filter. Separation of the plasma is achieved, and reinfusion of the cellular components then occurs. This technique performs well for specific plasma filtration scenarios but is reliant upon the filter pore size.[49-54]

Family-centered care is an integrated system of resources guided toward patient and family involvement and needs during hospitalization. The program should strive to provide family-centered care. A brief orientation to answer questions and set realistic goals and expectations is scheduled during the pretreatment phase. We focus on the family, clinical information, and supplemental teaching and support while the child is receiving treatment.

Family members are encouraged to get involved and actively participate in the care of their child.

The staff, in collaboration with the child life service, provides distractions and entertains the patient during treatment or any painful procedures. Board games, TVs, and reading materials are available to any child of different age groups. The health-care team in the PICU and apheresis program provides reassurance and comfort, as well as reinforcing the treatment regimen and protocols to the family and patient.

Specific Considerations for the ECMO Circuit

Apheresis is indicated when there is an acute clinical need to separate blood components. Therapeutic apheresis including total plasma exchange, red blood cell exchange, leukopheresis, and stem cell collection can be easily performed by the apheresis specialist during ECMO. A stopcock is placed on the venous line prebladder for the access of the withdrawal specimen. The returning line is placed downstream on the venous line, again preraceway. As all apheresis specialists managing the ECMO pump should be certified ECLS specialists, this procedure can be performed with relative ease, eliminating venous access (catheter) problems and alteration of total ECMO flow. The parallel apheresis circuit does not affect ECMO circuit flows. Once therapy is stabilized, the ECMO flows will remain unchanged. The initial "total" ECMO circuit compliance may transiently change during the initiation of apheresis. If the ECMO venous drainage is unrecognized as borderline or marginal, the bladder may chirp, suggesting an acute decrease in venous return. The servo regulation of the pump may also suddenly reduce ECMO flow. This may require an additional volume bolus during initiation of apheresis. The apheresis protocol and software from the manufacturer should be followed for continued maintenance of the separation therapy. Unique conditions may require the manual programming of the device or overriding specific parameters. The scope and nature of every unique scenario is beyond the scope of this manual, and when this occurs, it may be best to acquire additional expertise from the manufacturer or a more experienced center before beginning the therapy.

Responsibilities

- Verify procedure with apheresis / ECMO specialist, physician, and family.
- Assist in explaining indication, procedure, and risks to family.
- Record patient height, weight, hematocrit, and indication.

- Send baseline preprocedure labs CBC, Ica⁺, and electrolytes (notify physician of results).
- Labs for specific procedures (notify physician of results).
- TSM (red cell exchange).
- $CD_{34}+$, disease markers, and HIV (need consent) for stem cell harvest.
- Specific disease markers and HIV (need consent).
- Anti-inflammatory panels.
- Extra labs for multiple procedures (notify physician of results).
- Mg & Po4 & ICa⁺.
- PT/PTT.
- FDP, fibrinogen.
- IgG.
- Standby emergency replacement fluid (PRBCs, albumin, FFP, NS).
- Connect apheresis access line (using sterile and airless technique) to venous pigtail close to patient (prebladder).
- Connect apheresis return line (using sterile and airless technique) to any of the venous pigtails downstream from access line and preraceway.
- Halfway through procedure or if symptomatic for hypocalcaemia, send ICa⁺ (notify physician of results).
- Monitor ACTs. If apheresis decision to utilize citrate to bond calcium to prevent clotting in the pheresis, circuit adjustments in heparin may be necessary.
- If patient deteriorates, stop apheresis immediately, notify physician STAT, and follow ECLS protocol.
- When procedure is completed, disconnect apheresis access and return line (using sterile and airless technique) and flush pigtails with 1 cc NS and place port cap on site.
- Postprocedure send.
- ICa⁺, Mg⁺, electrolytes, and PT/PTT (notify physician of results).
- Anti-inflammatory panel.
- IgG.

Specific Humoral Considerations of Therapeutic Apheresis

Therapeutic plasma exchange (TPE) is a systemic immunomodulatory therapy. It removes specified plasma volumes and returns predetermined replacement fluids, most commonly plasma and/or albumin. The manipulation of removing, diluting, and returning foreign plasma components initiates an immune response, which can be seen in the elevation of all major circulating immune complexes one to three hours posttreatment. There is also serum elevation of complement, including C3a, C4a, and C5a, and an increase in the total number of circulating granulocytes and macrophages within the first two treatments. Lymphocytes increase in treatment 3, and the T helper/suppressor ratio increases in treatment 4. TPE involves cycling 100% of the patient's total blood volume, thereby removing putative pathologic material in the patient's plasma. The efficacy of treatment may be measured by a reduction in concentration of pathologic and toxic substances such as proinflammatory cytokines.[59, 62] The aggressive use of IgG concomitant with TPE has been widely reported for pretransplant patients and for blood group incompatibilities incurred with transplantation and rejection.[61-66] This should also be considered for all extended therapies due to the significant reduction of circulating immunoglobulins during repeated procedures. Circulating inflammatory mediators are widely recognized as contributing to the morbidity and mortality of certain clinical conditions. This is the predominant pathophysiology condition during sepsis, and the application of plasmapheresis has been directly shown to improve outcome and reduction of the "humoral" imbalance.[65-68] The direct filtration of these mediators has not been possible until the recent improvement in the biocompatibility of membranes. An immunoadsorption column with protein A covalently bound to a microprocessed silicone filter (Prosorba) has been historically utilized and may be added to the circuit in combination with TPE.[69] This greatly amplifies the immunomodulation of the extracorporeal circuit. The Prosorba column has been utilized to prevent graft versus host reactions in organ recipients and the reduction immunologic blood group incompatibilities in kidney transplant patients.[69] A polymixin B—immobilized fiber has also historically been used and has shown to significantly decrease circulating levels of endotoxin after TPE, but no study has shown a benefit to these absorptive therapies.[70]

Chapter 12

Physiology of Plasmapheresis

Physiologic Considerations

The clinical application of TPE begins with the age of the patient and the determination of the intravascular volume. Additional venous access is not necessary during ECMO. The type of priming fluid for the circuit is dependent on the patient's age. The older typical centrifuge circuits require 350 cc for priming and have a circuit volume of approximately 150 cc. The 18-kg child will have approximately a 12% dilution from the circuit, and this may be primed with blood to minimize the dilutional effects of priming. These packed blood cells will prevent further dilution of the hematocrit and anemia and for certain children, as well as possible hypovolemia.[69-75]

Smaller children are at greater risk, while larger children (> 20 kg) may tolerate priming with colloid or crystalloid. The choice of replacement fluids also varies depending on the diagnosis, indication, and/or institutional preference. The decision to utilize fresh frozen plasma or fractionated human albumin as priming and replacement fluid should be made clinically, based on the immunologic, protein, pulmonary, and cardiovascular condition of the child. Crystalloid solutions (normal saline) and colloid solutions (albumin or fresh frozen plasma) may be utilized alone or in combination. The risk of transfusion and physiologic complications increases with the use of foreign protein, but children with unstable or suboptimal physiology often benefit from the use of a combination of fresh frozen plasma and fractioned human albumin.[76-78]

Fresh frozen plasma is the replacement of choice if coagulation factors are depleted; however, administration requires immunologic compatibility and carries an increased risk of exposure to foreign protein. There are newer circuits primed with less than 100 cc and circulating less than 50 cc. These circuits may allow crystalloid priming for children greater than 8 kg.

TPE treatments are usually from one to three hours in duration. They may be ordered once a day or every other day for a period of three to four days. The number of treatments is dependent upon patient response and can usually be established after the completion of the first two treatments. Improved lab values and clinical status will become apparent for the rapid responder within the first twenty-four hours. Repeated therapies for conditions that are slowly responding should be cycled every four to seven treatments with a day or two without TPE. This will minimize the depletion of endogenous healthy circulating cofactors. Replacement of many cofactors may be carried out utilizing fresh frozen plasma and should be utilized for extended therapies. Specific cofactors may need to be measured and replaced as needed. Many centers routinely measure IgG levels and replace accordingly. Careful monitoring of inflammatory mediators, coagulation profiles, protein, and immunoglobulins will trace improvement and depletion of cofactors.

It is important to calculate the plasma volume to exchange. One-blood volume plasma exchange will exchange 63% of the circulating blood volume or toxin. A two-blood volume plasma exchange will remove 86%. Single-volume exchanges are typically performed, better tolerated, and successful when repeated after a day or two time delay. The series of repeated exchanges follows daily and every-other-day profiles. The typical total course for sepsis is four to ten treatments for sepsis. Many centers will increase this to fourteen treatments for sepsis, although the data is not available. The successful rapid responders will require five to seven treatments.[79]

We will institute a two-day holiday before proceeding with additional treatments for slow responders as all plasma—and protein-bound substances are readily removed during TPE and need to be reconstituted. The initial TPE calculation commonly recommends that a one and one half (1½) blood volume exchange is appropriate. Although many centers continue to perform single-volume exchanges for consecutive treatment, we perform 1½ volume exchanges throughout the TPE therapy for the sicker patients.

Cardiorespiratory

Sudden decreases in preload, acute changes in peripheral vascular resistance, and alteration of right ventricular compliance may occur from both the exposure to the extracorporeal circuit and volume shifting. The initiation of any extracorporeal circuit must take into consideration the underlying right and left ventricular lusitrophic and inotropic condition as well as the peripheral vascular resistance. Ventilated ECMO patients who are marginally preload dependent may suffer a decrease in pulmonary blood flow and left ventricular pressure. Larger patients generally respond to flow adjustments and volume replacement with protein containing solutions and rarely require inotropic support. Warming of the replacement fluids can help prevent complications such as hypothermia and "sickling" in susceptible patients. There is no evidence of a primary change in pulmonary compliance and no evidence of alteration in gas exchange, but there may be a sudden change in peripheral vascular resistance from exposure to foreign surfaces usually amenable to volume infusion. There may be an improvement in left ventricular function after therapy with the reduction of circulating mediators, seen more commonly in gram-negative sepsis.[65,70,75]

Metabolic

The most frequently encountered electrolyte disturbances and complication results from abnormalities in the soluble calcium, when citrate is used as an additional anticoagulant. Hypocalcaemia is most frequently seen in patients with severe liver dysfunction, those receiving citrated fresh frozen plasma, or during procedures with a high citrate-blood ratio.[77-79]

Children should also be observed for complications of hyperkalemia. Depletion of plasma proteins, especially coagulation factors, and immunologic factors may occur if repeated procedures are required. Prevention and management of hypocalcaemia includes administration of supplemental calcium (gluconate or chloride). Monitoring of pH, serum protein, and the reduction in all-circulating enzymes during a prolonged manipulation of intravascular components is important.

Hematological

High blood flow rates may create hemolysis if the circuit is twisted or kinked. Significant hemolysis may precipitate DIC or mimic a transfusion reaction. Hemolysis may be detected by monitoring the plasma color. Monitoring of hemoglobin, hematocrit, platelets, and coagulation factors such as PT/PTT, fibrinogen, and FDP are also essential for evaluation of the hematological status. There may be a shifting of the ACTs as well. A decrease in circulating immunoglobulins or coagulation cofactors may be addressed by the infusion of fresh frozen plasma, IgG, fibrinogen, or factor VII. Hemodilution with unwarmed fluids may promote hypothermia.

Circuit Priming

The fluid status of the patient needs to be carefully evaluated. The goal is usually to leave the patient in a fluid balance range of no more than 75%-125% of calculated baseline. The Cobe Spectra machine default volume level is 100% baseline (no net increase or decrease). Crystalloid prime is often used for children larger than 45 kg. Colloid prime is recommended for children 20-45 kg. The physician may order blood prime for any child. Children less than 20 kg often require one unit of donor-compatible CMV negative, irradiated, leukodepleted blood to prime the apheresis circuit. The methods of blood priming will be dependent on the physician's clinical decision. Blood priming with reconstituted blood is often chosen when the hematocrit is desired to be normal or high. Anemia, volume-overloaded, or volume-intolerant patients may require packed RBCs when priming. Clinically stable children often tolerate either solution.

A Cobe Spectra circuit requires 345 cc to prime. The circulating internal volume is 150 cc, and the rinse-back volume is 195 cc. If rinse back is given when the procedure is programmed to leave the patient at 100% balance, then the patient will be 195 cc positive at the end of the procedure. One should not rinse back at end of a procedure unless there is a need to increase the patient's volume. The recorded values can be subtracted from final-run values to measure total volume given.

Calculation of Fluid Balance

(replacement rate + AC rate) × 100 plasma flow rate

When blood priming with reconstituted whole blood to a desired hematocrit the formula is this:

$$\text{Volume of RBC post dilution} = \frac{(\text{Hct RBC from banked blood bag}) \times (\text{vol. RBC bag})}{(\text{desired Hct for prime})}$$

- The volume of diluent to add to PRBC bag = total vol. RBC after dilution—initial vol. PRBC bag.
- The volume of RBCs after dilution = volume of diluent—volume of initial PRBCs.
- The diluent may be a combination of FFP, 5% albumin, or normal saline.

Example

RBC Hct = 70%
RBC volume = 220 mL.
Desired Hct for prime = 30%
Volume of RBC unit after dilution = (0.70) × (220 mL.) = 513 mL.
Volume of diluent = 513 mL.—220 mL. = 293 mL.
Add 293 cc of fluid to the original unit of PRBCs to achieve a desired Hct of 30%.

- When blood priming with packed red blood cells, the machine should be programmed with the Hct of PRBCs in the banked blood bag.
- When the blood prime reaches the return saline manifold during the initiation of the procedure, record the volume-processed at that point, at the anticoagulant (AC) inlet plasma.
- This volume may be replaced if applicable.
- Plasma processed from prime is added to the target value so that this amount will correct the run so that the desired patient blood product is removed.

Anticoagulation

- Anticoagulation (AC) is initiated to minimize clotting of the blood as it travels through the circuit.
- The most frequently used anticoagulant is citrate.
- The most common form of citrate used is ACD-A.
- Most of the ACD-A is processed from the circuit when exposed to the calcium in the circuit.
- Each 100 mL of ACD-A contains
    o 2.2 g of sodium citrate (hydrous)
    o 730 mg citric acid (anhydrous)
    o 2.45 g dextrose (anhydrous)
- The infusion rate for AC is dependent on the total blood volume and type of replacement fluid (mL of AC/min/liter) of total blood volume.
- The spectra control program will minimize the citrate reactions by adjusting this flow rate.
- The clinical condition may alternatively require the use of heparin.
- Heparin binds antithrombin III and blocks clotting factor activity of VII, IX, X, XI, XII.
- The use of heparin requires the monitoring of clotting times.

- A convenient bedside determination of in vivo clotting is the measurement of an activated clotting time (ACT).
- An accepted range for ACTs utilizing the I-stat technique is 130-150 without ECMO.
- The ECMO patient generally requires increased anticoagulation (ACT 160-180).
- The entire "circuit" should be managed according to the ECMO patient's needs.
- The heparin should be infused directly into the circuit to maintain anticoagulation of the circuit.

Complications

One of the earliest pediatric programs began in 1994 and has provided care to over 300 patients with over 1,200 procedures.[79] Clinical events that required intervention occurred in 47 percent (47%) of our treatments with one fatality. Decreased blood pressure was noted in 5.6%, increased blood pressure at 3.5 %, and hypocalcaemia at 11%. Noninterventional events (nausea, vomiting, increased heart rate, tingling) occurred in 6.2% of patients.[79] Other complications of vascular access included hematoma at the site of catheter insertion, pneumo/hemothorax, retroperitoneal bleed, infection, thrombosis, and air embolism.

Hypocalcaemia is the most frequent complication. The contributing factor is citrate anticoagulant in the PRBC bag and ACD-A. The patient may complain of tingling/numbness of lips, fingers or toes; at times, they may also feel lightheaded or dizzy. In cases of severe hypocalcaemia, the patient can develop a dysrrhythmia. The calcium in the blood binds to the ACD, causing gradual depletion of the circulating calcium. Electrolytes are monitored before, during, and after each procedure with special emphasis on magnesium, ionized calcium, and potassium levels. For procedures more than an hour in length, the calcium levels must be monitored every hour until the end of the procedure. Calcium gluconate drips can be infused throughout lengthy treatments. As an emergent response to arrhythmias, it is recommended to stop the procedure and administer IV calcium chloride. If the calcium level is within normal limits, the procedure can be resumed with ongoing calcium monitoring. The management of hypocalcaemia includes slowing down the inlet flow (20 cc/min), sending a stat-ionized calcium and giving calcium replacements such as calcium chloride 10% (20-25 mg/kg/dose) and calcium gluconate 100-500 mg/kg/d continuous drip in four divided doses.

Coagulation abnormalities are commonly twofold. First is a depletion of coagulation factors as they are removed during TPE. This can be compounded by the fact that albumin, or any replacement fluid that does not contain coagulation factors, will add a dilutional effect to the serum. Recovery of coagulation factors is characterized by a rapid four-hour increase and a slower rise in circulating cofactors during the next twenty-four hours after a single exchange. When multiple treatments are performed over a short period (three or more treatments per week), the depletion in clotting factors is more pronounced and may require several days for spontaneous recovery.[77] By using fresh frozen plasma as a replacement fluid, the risks of iatrogenic hemodilution of circulating coagulation cofactors can be minimized. There is an increased risk of using human products that should always be considered.[78]

Transfusion Reaction—Contributing factors include ABO mismatch (not following blood bank protocol) and multiple transfusions. Prevention includes administration of leukodepleted blood product and premedication of sensitive patients. Patients that receive multiple treatments or transfusions may have a better response if an antihistamine is administered before treatment. When a transfusion reaction occurs, the procedure is discontinued, and instituted transfusion reaction protocols are followed. Maintain perfusion by giving crystalloids and osmotic diuretics. Check urine for hemolysis.[46] Thrombocytopenia can result from loss of platelets in the discarded plasma during dilution or via filter thrombosis. There is a greater loss of platelets using the centrifugal method than by membrane plasma separation. Wood and Jacobs (1986) have also shown decreases in the hematocrit by 10% after each plasmapheresis treatment in the absence of any extracorporeal losses or hemolysis.

Hypothermia—Contributing factors are due to the circuit, the use of cold/cool replacement fluids, and patient size. It is also due to the rapid loss of circulating volume that patients may experience chills or shivering. Preventive measures include using warmed replacement fluids. Slowing down the inlet flow may improve hypothermia. It may help to also warm to the infusing replacement fluid via circuit warmer.

CHAPTER 13

Nursing and Plasmapheresis

Patient Nursing Care of ECMO TPE Patient

Full explanation and understanding is essential prior to the insertion of the venous access device as well as the actual apheresis procedure. Providing the patient and family with written materials about the purpose and benefits of the TPE procedure and allowing time to answer any questions or concerns before beginning the procedure promotes a better environment. Informed consent for the line placement, blood products, and procedure is standard.

Orders

- Type of procedure, replacement fluid, volume to be processed, and ending fluid balance should all be checked and verified.
- The patient's height, weight, and gender are important for programming the machine.
- The baseline labs include a CBC, ionized calcium (ICA), electrolytes, Mg, PO4, PT, PTT (for multiple runs). Vital signs include EKG, temperature, B/P, and O_2 saturation.
- A detailed medication history is required.
- Continuous cardiac and O_2 saturation monitoring monitor of all ECMO patients must occur during the procedure. Blood pressure and heart rate are recorded at least every fifteen minutes.
- Some patients require premedication with Solu-Medrol or Benadryl.
- Sedation and pain medication should be monitored during this plasma dilution and replacement.

- During the treatment, the patient must be monitored for signs of hypocalcaemia, hypotension, hypothermia, or any signs of possible additional transfusion reactions.
- The ionized calcium is repeated at least one hour or midway into the procedure if citrate is infused.
- After the procedure, ICa^+, CBC, Mg^+, and PO_4^{-2} are measured.
- If the patient requires multiple treatments, protein, IgG, coagulation factors, and PT/PTT are measured.
- Plasma/protein-bound medications may also be removed during apheresis.
- A clinical assessment of the patient should be performed at the start of every procedure and includes vital signs, neurological status, and the extracorporeal circuit.
- The date and time of initiation of treatment must be recorded.
- The effluent, color or texture of fluids, and any mechanical problems during treatment are recorded.
- Documentation should also include
  o fluid replacement used,
  o change in patient status during treatment,
  o any intervention,
  o date and time of end of treatment, and
  o patient tolerance to treatment.
- Pretreatment labs and labs drawn during the treatment should also be recorded. Family understanding and participation should also be documented.

Chapter 14

Apheresis Specialist Training and Competencies

An outline of our recommendations and guidelines to certify individuals as apheresis specialists upon successful completion of the following three modules:

Module I—Didactic—The apheresis specialist candidate will complete thirty-two hours of didactic lectures. These hours will include a formal lecture program. Upon completion of these hours, a written test will be given. A passing score of 85% must be achieved.

Module II—Water Labs—The apheresis specialist candidate will complete eight hours of supervised water lab training plus a final test of emergency drills. This does not include individual practice sessions that are required in order to pass the final test. These practice hours will vary according to the individual's skill level but will not be less than four hours.

Module III—Clinical Orientation—The apheresis specialist candidate will complete a minimum of thirty-six hours of clinical orientation. Upon completion of these hours, the nurse manager and extracorporeal coordinator of the ECLS team will review the skills checklists. If any skill requirements have not been met, further bedside orientation may be warranted.

Recertification—Emergency water lab check off four times annually. Didactic and/or practical continuing education in the form of lectures, workshops, or animal laboratory experience of not less than eight (8) hours per year.

Planned Maintenance, Calibration Testing, and Procedure for Equipment Failure

The performance of all medical equipment is tested according to relevant standards by the clinical engineering department. A planned maintenance program and calibration testing that assures the accuracy and the clinical engineering department in collaboration with the apheresis section must establish longevity of the system. All calibration and maintenance testing is based on the recommendation of the manufacturer.

In the event of equipment failure, notification to the service dispatch promptly occurs. The repair response is required within twenty-four hours. Once repair is completed, notification to the clinical engineering department is issued, and all service repairs documentation is sent to the clinical engineering department for safekeeping and tracking.

Apheresis Checklist

Patient's Name:_____Date: _____
Reviewed by Medical Director or Designee Date:_____Signature:_____
Account #:_____
Apheresis Specialist_____

Date/Notes	Done	Procedure
		1. Pheresis consult obtained. a. Attending notified.

		2. Appropriate staff notified.
		    a. Fellow on call.
		    b. Nurse Manager/CNS

		3. Family provided with apheresis brochure, indications, risks, procedure, and understanding of participation is documented.

			4. Preapheresis criteria met: a. Informed consent /blood transfusion consent obtained b. Appropriate labs reviewed and parameters met c. CBC with diff. (platelets > 50,000, Hgb > 8, Hct > 24) d. PT, PTT (< 13—≤ 35) e. Ionized calcium (≥ 1.0) f. If patient is less than 18 kg, do type and crossmatch and sent to blood bank (request Hct on bag).
			3. Labs reviewed by physician and apheresis specialist (H/H, PT, PTT, ICa⁺); corrective action taken before procedure
			4. Patient is prepared for apheresis treatment a. Physician / apheresis specialist evaluates patient (including height [cm], weight [kg], and temperature) b. History/physical/medication assessment done c. Patient/family teaching reinforced; consent reviewed; documented in medical record d. Patient sedation reviewed for procedure e. Machine primed and ready for use
			8. Patient's prepheresis condition reviewed and documented; pheresis started.

		9. Reassessment/document (midprocedure) by physician and specialist:
		   a. sedation status
		   b. neuro status
		   c. vital signs
		   d. treatment tolerance
		   f. evidence of hypocalcemia

		11. Patient's condition reviewed and documented postprocedure including the following:
		   a. sedation status
		   b. neuro status
		   c. vital signs
		   e. tolerance of procedure

		12. Two hours postcompletion, obtain CBC and ionized CA^+
		13. Procedure and condition reviewed with family and documented in medical record
		14. Quality clinical indicators documented
		15. Case reviewed by medical director, nurse manager, and team
		16. Quality process control continued

Chapter 15

ECMO Certification

ECMO Specialist Competencies

The ECMO center will certify individuals as ECMO specialist upon successful completion of the following five modules. This certification is based upon recommended guidelines from the ELSO organization.

Module I—Didactic

The ECMO specialist candidate will complete thirty-two hours of didactic lectures. These hours will include a formal lecture program. Upon completion of these hours, a written test will be given. A passing score of 85% must be achieved.

Module II—Water Labs

The ECMO specialist candidate will complete twenty-four hours of supervised water lab training plus a final test of emergency drills. This does not include individual practice sessions, which are required in order to pass the final test. These practice hours will vary according to the individual's skill level but will not be less than ten hours.

Module III—Animal Labs

The ECMO specialist candidate will complete a minimum of eight hours of clinical animal laboratory experience. Specific goals as outlined in the

ECMO protocol must be met at each animal lab. In the event that these goals are not met, additional animal labs may need to be scheduled.

Module IV—Clinical Orientation

The ECMO specialist candidate will complete a minimum of sixty hours of clinical orientation. Upon completion of these hours, the nurse manager and extracorporeal specialist of the ECMO team will review the skills checklists. If any skill requirements have not been met, further bedside orientation may be warranted.

ECMO Specialist Commitment

Recertification—Annual

1. An emergency water lab check off four times annually.
2. Didactic and/or practical continuing education in the form of lectures, workshops, or animal laboratory experience of not less than eight (8) hours per year. Programs must be approved by the ECMO program.

ECMO Specialist Training Program—Educational Goals

Module I—Didactic

The ECMO specialist candidate will be able to

1. describe the pathophysiology of the newborn ECMO candidate;
2. describe criteria for choosing a neonatal ECMO candidate, including precluding disease states;
3. describe criteria for choosing a pediatric ECMO candidate, including cardiac, respiratory, and septic criteria;
4. discuss the hemodynamics of perfusion on various organ systems;
5. describe the concepts of oxygen delivery and consumption;
6. describe the mechanisms of anticoagulation as related to the ECMO circuit;
7. describe the ventilatory support mechanisms for a patient on ECMO;
8. interpret a blood gas result and discuss appropriate interventions;
9. interpret various laboratory results, their relationship to ECMO, and their treatment modalities;

10. describe the mechanisms of flow and sweep as related to the ECMO circuit;
11. describe the ECMO specialist's role in the cannulation, idling, and decannulation procedures;
12. describe the mechanisms involved in a trial-off period;
13. list three possible complications of an ECMO patient;
14. discuss how to troubleshoot any patient problem that may arise;
15. describe the nursing interventions as related to the ECMO patient;
16. discuss hemofiltration, its setup procedure, and precautions when used during ECMO;
17. discuss the indications for veno-venous ECMO; and
18. discuss oxygen delivery in veno-venous ECMO.

Module II—Water Labs

The ECMO specialist candidate will be able to

1. describe the components to the ECMO circuit, including the equipment and disposables;
2. describe and perform how to troubleshoot a malfunctioning piece of equipment;
3. set up and crystalloid prime the ECMO circuit as per ECMO protocol;
4. demonstrate each of the emergency drills with appropriate interventions as outlined in the ECMO protocol in a timely manner;
5. describe and perform the proper procedure for removing a patient from bypass;
6. describe and perform the proper procedure for placing a patient on bypass;
7. describe the proper personnel that should be present in the event of an emergency;
8. demonstrate knowledge of the items in the ECMO supply room;
9. describe the role of each person involved in an emergency;
10. demonstrate appropriate aseptic/sterile technique;
11. describe the circuit changes necessary to change from veno-venous ECMO to veno-arterial ECMO; and
12. describe coming on and off bypass and weaning during veno-venous ECMO.

Module III—Clinical Orientation

The ECMO specialist candidate will be able to

1. demonstrate appropriate hand-washing procedure;
2. give a detailed report to an oncoming ECMO specialist;
3. appropriately assess the ECMO circuit as per ECMO protocol;
4. perform an ACT as per ECMO protocol;
5. troubleshoot an erroneous ACT accordingly;
6. demonstrate proper blood gas sampling technique from the ECMO circuit;
7. demonstrate the calibration procedure for the Oximetrix computer;
8. demonstrate proper technique in blood sampling from the ECMO circuit;
9. document appropriately on all ECMO records;
10. properly check blood product supplies and record blood refrigerator temperature;
11. properly administer blood products into the ECMO circuit and properly document such products on the ECMO flow sheet;
12. prepare the heparin drip as per ECMO protocol and administer it to the circuit;
13. change "sticky" stopcocks as required per ECMO protocol;
14. describe the relationship of flow-to-oxygen delivery;
15. describe the relationship of sweep-to-CO_2 removal;
16. discuss cardiopulmonary physiology of the ECMO patient;
17. interpret an ABG and discuss appropriate interventions as related to ECMO;
18. interpret lab results and discuss appropriate interventions as related to ECMO;
19. interpret venous saturation readings and discuss appropriate interventions as related to ECMO;
20. assess clinical status of the ECMO patient, including vital signs and possible clinical interventions;
21. describe the proper procedure for the dressing change to the cannula site and appropriate interventions for hemorrhage;
22. perform appropriate emergency ECMO adjustments during clinical changes;
23. discuss the contents of the ECMO cart and properly restock it;
24. perform estimation of oxygen delivery, oxygen consumption, and maximum flow;

25. demonstrate proper technique in adjusting flow, sweep, and heparin drip;
26. demonstrate the specialist's responsibility during cannulation and decannulation;
27. demonstrate the specialist's responsibility during a trial-off period;
28. demonstrate proper maintenance and cleanliness of all ECMO equipment;
29. demonstrate proper procedure during any emergency that may arise;
30. demonstrate knowledge of items in the ECMO supply room;
31. demonstrate communication skills when relating to parents and medical staff;
32. discuss use of pulmonary function testing in relationship to using ECMO; and
33. discuss recirculation physiology and calculation during veno-venous ECMO.

Chapter 16

Final Clinical Water Lab 1

Name :_____Date: _____
Evaluator:_____

1. **Gas Source Failure**

    a. **Oxygen Failure**

    ____Blender will alarm and deliver 100% air
    ____Check all connections and other wall sources
    ____Remove tubing from blender and attach to oxygen transport tank
    ____Notify respiratory of tank need

Comments:

   b. **Air Failure**

    ____Blender will alarm and deliver 100% oxygen
    ____Bypass blender by using flowmeter directly in wall

Comments:

2. **Flow Display Failure—Cobe**

    ____No digital display with pump on and tubing ID button pushed
    ____Push RPM display button; if it works, use stroke volume formula flow = RPMs × 13 mL (Cobe)

____If there is still no display, calculate flow as follows:

- Place tape on one roller head
- Count revolutions in ten (10) seconds
- Multiply by six (6)
- Use stroke volume formula

Comments:

3. Heater Failure

____Use backup heater
____Turn up settings on ECMO radiant warmer bed

Comments:

4. Power Failure

____Call ECMO physician
____Do not hand crank in the dark if you can't see the bladder
____Turn off the power switch
____Turn down the speed knob
____Place hand crank in hole
____Place hand on bladder
____Turn hand crank *counterclockwise* while continually watching bladder
____Count revolutions over ten (10) seconds to determine speed or monitor venous saturations
____Do not chart anything at this time

Comments:

5. Pump Failure

____Call ECMO physician
____If possible, hand crank
____Have someone get the backup pump from the storage room
____Have them plug in the pump
____Call ECMO physician, emergency vent settings
____Come off bypass as per protocol
____Remove tubing from pump
____Push old pump out of the way

____Place tubing in pump and set a gross occlusion with clamp on the positive side of the pump head
____Turn on the bladder box alarms and recirculate
____Go on bypass as per protocol
____Recirculate, checking for air, clamps, etc.
____Once patient is stable, have ECMO coordinator or ECMO priming specialist come in and set fine occlusion
____Check ACT, pump gases immediately

Comments:

6. Cracked Stopcock

____Clamp pigtail with tubing clamp wrapped in two by twos
____Remove stopcock and replace
____Aspirate air and flush

Comments:

7. Damaged Pigtail

____Clamp pigtail immediately if leaking
____Prepare new pigtail, notify ECMO physician
____Emergency vent setting
____Come off bypass as per protocol
____Clamp tubing on both sides of pigtail
____Remove old pigtail and replace with new one, making an airless connection
____Remove clamp that opens system to bladder
____Remove clamps and recirculate
____Go on bypass as per protocol
____Check ACT, pump gases

Comments:

8. Wear in Raceway Tubing

Advance tubing out of raceway to the positive side of the pump as follows:

____Mark tubing near inlet and outlet tubing clamp
____Notify ECMO physician, emergency vent settings

____Come off bypass as per protocol
____Shut off power to pump
____Remove tubing from raceway and move to positive if possible
____Place tubing back in raceway
____Recirculate and check circuit
____Go back on bypass as per protocol
____When patient is stable, have ECMO coordinator or ECMO priming specialist set fine occlusion
____Check ACT, pump gases

Comments:

9. **Raceway Tubing Rupture**

   ____Notify ECMO physician, emergency vent settings
   ____Come off bypass as per protocol
   ____Shut off power to pump
   ____Supplies
   - ____Super Tygon raceway tubing
   - ____Two ¼ × ¼ or 3/8 × 3/8 connectors
   - ____ER kit
   - ____Clamps

   ____Place clamps on each side of tubing that was in raceway
   ____Remove tubing
   ____Cut out raceway using Betadine swabs and number 10 blade or sterile scissors
   ____Remove new tubing from package and place connectors on each end
   ____Connect new tubing on inlet side and prime with crystalloid
   ____Make airless connection to distal end
   ____Place tubing back in roller head, set a gross occlusion
   ____Recirculate
   ____Go back on bypass as per protocol
   ____Check ACT, pump gases
   ____When patient is stable, have ECMO coordinator or ECMO priming specialist set fine occlusion

Comments:

10. **Hole in Tubing**

    ____Call ECMO physician, emergency vent settings

____Come off bypass if in main circuit
____Clamp one inch proximal and distal to hole
____Swab with Betadine and cut tubing through defect, or if large, cut out defective tubing
____Place ¼ × ¼ connector on one end of tubing (or 3/8 × 3/8 or ½ × ½ connector)
____Fill connector with flush and make airless connection to other end
____Remove clamps and recirculate
____Go back on bypass as per protocol
____Check ACT, ABGs

Comments:

11. Connector Separation

____Call ECMO physician, emergency vent settings
____Come off bypass as per protocol
____Clamp loose tubing
____Refill line with flush and reconnect
____If connection is very loose, cut off end of tubing
____Look for cause of tubing separation
____Remove clamps and recirculate to remove air
____Go back on bypass as per protocol
____Double tie band connections
____Check ACT, ABGs

Comments:

12. Air in Circuit

Prebladder

____Remove through bladder

Oxygenator

____Remove through sampling port on top of oxygenator

Heat exchanger

____Call ECMO physician, emergency vent settings

____Come off bypass as per protocol
____Walk air back to platelet infusion pigtail
____Withdraw slowly with syringe
____Recirculate and go back on bypass as per protocol
____Check ACT, ABGs

Arterial Line

____Call ECMO physician, emergency vent settings
____Come off bypass immediately
____Recirculate through bridge
____Walk any air in cannulae back to patient bridge
____Go back on bypass as per protocol check
____ACT, ABGs

Patient Bridge

____If not on venous side of clamp, walk back down to bladder and remove
____If on arterial side of clamp, place second clamp on the other side of the air and remove first clamp and remove as before

Comments:

13. Decannulation

Venous Decannulation

____Call ECMO physician, emergency vent settings
____Clamp prebladder
____Continue infusing through arterial line to maintain pressure by adding volume to bladder
____Tighten tourniquet if left in
____Have available person place pressure on site until surgeon is present

Arterial Decannulation

____Call ECMO physician, emergency vent settings
____Come off bypass as per protocol
____Tighten tourniquet if available

___Place pressure
___Clamp postbladder
___Retrograde infuse by adding volume to bladder box, unclamping venous cannula to maintain pressure
___Be sure patient bridge is clamped

Comments:

14. Clots in the Circuit

___If clots are seen anywhere other than the bladder, check the entire circuit for clots
___If clots are only in bladder, try to withdraw with syringe; otherwise, leave them alone, unless clot is near outlet, change out bladder
___If clots are found in the patient bridge, do not flush and change it out like the raceway tubing
___Clots found distal to the oxygenator require a complete circuit change

Comments:

15. Oxygenator Failure

Diagnosis

___Leaks identified by blood dripping from gas outlet
___If less than 30 mL/hr by three-hour measure and replace mL/mL
___Maintain ACTs 160-180 seconds
___Administer platelets to raise level to 150,000
___Check premembrane and postmembrane pressures every four (4) hours
___Check gas outlet port for obstruction every thirty (30) minutes
___If it becomes obstructed, change out oxygenator
___Watch for increased CO_2 and decreased pO_2 (CO_2 first!)
___Watch transmembrane pressures; when pressure drop is 100 mmHg greater than baseline readings at the same extracorporeal flow, change the oxygenator
___When patient gases abruptly change, check transfer to determine if oxygenator failure is present

O_2 Transfer for Medtronic 0800 = 60-70 mL O_2/m^2/minute
AV O_2 transfer =
$$\frac{(CaO_2 - CvO_2)(1.36 \times Hgb) \times 10 \times flow}{100\%}$$

Comments:

16. Heat Exchanger Failure

a. Leak identification

    ____Water to blood leak
    ____Hemolysis
    ____Decreased Hgb
    ____Increased K
    ____Acidosis
    ____Increased volume
    ____Blood to water leak
    ____Pink water in lines
    ____Blood exiting vents

Comments:

b. **Disconnecting Bypass**

    ____If leak is noted, turn off heater first
    ____Then drain exchanger
    ____Call ECMO physician, emergency vent settings
    ____Come off bypass immediately
    ____Double clamp 2" from heat exchanger inlet and outlet
    ____Cut out old heat exchanger
    ____Reconnect inlet and outlet lines with a ¼" × ¼" connector; make an airless connection
    ____Recirculate to remove any air
    ____Go back on bypass, increase temp setting on ECMO radiant warmer
    ____Check ACT, ABG

Comments:

Final Clinical Water Lab II

Name: _____ Date:_____
Evaluator:_____

Inappropriate Venous Return

____Palpation of the venous line can show position versus volume problems
____Elevate the patient as high as possible

Comments:

2. **Bladder Box Function**

____Diagnose if the bladder is too sensitive
____Test the bladder box function by clamping the venous line
____If inadequate flow persists with proper bladder box function, change the diameter of the venous drainage line
____Standby alarms
____Wiring the pump
____Shimming the bladder can decrease bladder sensitivity

Comments:

3. **Raceway Calculations**

____If the RPMs are greater than 100 rpm, change the raceway to the appropriate size
____If the raceway positioning is a problem, open the pump outlet and let the tubing find its natural curve
____A raceway segment can be used 144 hours; after this time, the raceway must be walked

Comments:

4. **Oxygenator Pressure Monitoring**

____Measure preoxygenator and postoxygenator pressures with the same monitor

Comments:

5. **Serum Hemoglobin**

    ____Shows destruction of red blood cells
    ____Can be caused by clots in the circuit or overocclusion of the roller pump
    ____Normal is 0; all patients will have some hemolysis
    ____Daily monitoring for acute changes

Comments:

6. **Hemofiltration**

    ____Flows from preoxygenator to prebladder
    ____Calculate the actual ECMO flow when the filter is open
    ____Hemofiltration with dialysis
    ____Pump *in* volume + ordered diuresis = pump *out* volume
    ____Requires double ultrafiltrate ports
    ____Follow hemodialysis orders when appropriate

Comments:

7. **Transonic Flowmeter**

    ____Anytime actual flow is needed
    ____Must be used on appropriate wall thickness PVC tubing
    ____Transonic jelly must be squirted into the tubing channel before attaching
    ____If the monitor reads negative numbers, press the invert button
    ____Calibration should be done daily by clamping input and output tubing around probe then zeroing meter

Comments:

8. **In Vivo Roller Pump Occlusion**

    Shopping List

    ____Two-foot PVC monitoring line
    ____Stopcock

____Sodium chloride
____60 mL syringe
____6 mL syringe

Procedure

____Preprime monitor line with sodium chloride
____Attach two-foot monitor line with stopcock and 6 mL syringe to ACT sample port
____Open the ACT sample port and aspirate air from the monitor line
____Close stopcock
____Connect 60 mL syringe to bladder port
____Come off bypass, pump off then vein-bridge-artery
____Emergency ventilator settings
____Clamp preoxygenator, post ACT sample site
____Clamp prebladder
____Set rollers at nine and three
____Totally occlude tubing with roller thumb wheel
____Withdraw blood/fluid into the 60 mL syringe until the bladder controller alarms
____Silence bladder controller alarms
____Hold stopcock and monitor line level with the top of the oxygenator
____Open stopcock on top of the monitor line
____Watch column of fluid in the monitor line; it should **not** move
____Deocclude raceway one click at a time, watching for fluid column to fall in monitor line
____Deocclude until fluid movement is consistent (no stopping)
____Close stopcock on top of the monitor line
____Turn off the ACT sample site
____Reinfuse the volume in the 60 mL syringe back into the bladder
____Remove prebladder clamp
____Remove preoxygenator clamp
____Circuit check
____Go back on bypass per protocol (artery-bridge-vein)
____Reactivate alarms on Seabrook bladder controller
____Remove the two-foot monitor line

ABBREVIATION LIST

A	Arterial
ABG	Arterial blood gas
ACT	Activated clotting time (in seconds)
AGA	Appropriate for gestational age
ATN	Acute tubular necrosis
B	Bridge
BPD	Bronchopulmonary dysplasia
BW	Birth weight
CBG	Capillary blood gas
CHD	Congenital heart disease
CDH	Congenital diaphragmatic hernia
CPAP	Continuous positive airway pressure
CPIP	Continuous pulmonary insufficiency of prematurity
CNS	Central nervous system
CT	Chest tube
CXR	Chest x-ray
ECMO	Extracorporeal membrane oxygenation
EDC	Estimated date of confinement
HMD	Hyaline membrane disease (RDS)
ICH	Intracranial hemorrhage
LGA	Large for gestational age
L/C	Lecithin sphingomyelin ratio (test of fetal maturity)
MAS	Meconium aspiration syndrome
NEC	Necrotizing enterocolitis
NSVD	Normal spontaneous vaginal delivery
PDA	Patent ductus arteriosus
PFO	Patent foramen ovale
PIE	Pulmonary interstitial emphysema

PPHN	Persistent pulmonary artery hypertension
PROM	Premature rupture of membranes
PT	Pneumothorax
RDS	Respiratory distress syndrome
RLF	Retrolental fibroplasia
RR	Respiratory rate
SGA	Small for gestational age
TEF	Tracheo-esophageal fistula
TTN	Transient tachypnea of the newborn
UAC	Umbilical arterial catheter
U/S	Ultrasound
UVC	Umbilical venous catheter
V	Venous
VRM	Venous return monitor

BIBLIOGRAPHY

1. Ni Maoshing, The Yellow Emperor's Classic of Medicine, Shambhala Publications, Inc. 1995
2. http://www.britannica.com/EBchecked/topic/23162/Anaximenes-Of-Miletus
3. **Hippocrates. *Apanta ta tou IppokratouV*.** *Omnia opera Hippocratis.* Venice: Aldus Manutius, 1526. http://www.nlm.nih.gov/hmd/greek/greek_rationality.html
4. http://www.britannica.com/EBchecked/topic/145475/Ctesibius-Of-Alexandria
5. http://science.jrank.org/pages/10147/Medicine-in-India-Systematic-Medicine.html">Medicine in India—Systematic Medicine</a>
6. http://en.wikipedia.org/wiki/Pneumatic_chemistry
7. Lower R, *Tractatus_de_corde:_item_de_motu_&_colore_sanguinis_et_chyli_in_eum transitu*. Londini: Typis Jo Redmayne, impensis Jacobi Allestry, 1669, [KCSMD Historical Collection QP111.4 LOW], http://www.pbs.org/wnet/redgold/innovators/bio_lower2.html#13
8. WM. Deb. Macnider, National Academy of Sciences of the United States of America, Biographical Memoirs, vol. XXIV—sixth memoir, presented to the Academy at the Annual Meeting, 1946
9. Abel JJ, Roundtree LG, Turner BB: On the removal of diffusible substances from the circulating blood by means of dialysis. *Trans Assoc Am Physicians* 28: 51, 1913
10. Kolff WJ, Berk HThJ, Ter Welle M, Van Der Ley AJW, Van Dyk EC, Noordwijk J. The artificial kidney: A dialyzer with a great area. Acta Med Scand 117:120, 1944
11. Kambic HE, Nose Y. Historical perspective on plasmapheresis. Therapeutic Apheresis, 1997. 1:83-108.

12. W.J. Kolff, ARTIFICIAL ORGANS FORTY YEARS AND BEYOND http://www.stanford.edu/dept/HPS/transplant/html/kolff.html
13. Kolf WJ, Effler DB, Groves LK, Peereboom G, Moraca PP, Disposable membrane oxygenator (heart-lung) machine and it's use ini experimental surgery, Cleve Clin Q 1956; 23:67-97
14. Gibbon JH, Application of a mechanical heart lung apparatus to cardiac surgery. Minn Med 1954; 37:171-185
15. Clowes GH Jr., Hopkins AL., Neville WE. An artificial lung dependent upon diffusion of oxygen and carbon dioxide through plastic membranes, Journal of Thoracic Surgery. 32(5):630-7, 1956 Nov.
16. Lillehei CW. History of the development of extracorporeal circulation. 1st ed. Boston: Blackwell Scientific Publications; 1993
17. Adams WS. Skoog WA. The management of multiple myeloma, Journal of Chronic Diseases. 6(4):446-56, 1957 Oct
18. Hill JD, O'Brien TG, Murray JJ, et.al. Prolonged extracorporeal oxygenation for acute post-traumatic respiratory failure (shock-lung syndrome) Use of the Bramson membrane lung, N. Engl J Med 1972; 286:629-634.
19. Zapol WM, Snider MT, Hill JD et al. Extracorporeal membrane oxygenation in severe acute respiratory distress. JAMA 1979; 242:2193-2196.
20. Bartlett RH Esperanza. Presidential Address. Trans. Am. Soc. Artif. Organs, 1985;31:723-726.
21. Bartlett Rh, Andrews AF, Toomasian JM, Haiduc NJ, Gazzaniga AB. Extracorporeal membrane oxygenation for newborn respiratory failure; forty-five cases. Surgery 1982; 92:425-433
22. Extracorporeal Life Support Organization, Ann Arbor Michigan, Registry July 2011, http://www.elso.med.umich.edu/Default.htm
23. Mitchell DG, Merton DA, Graziani, LJ. Desai HJ, Desai SA, Wolfson PJ, Gross GW., Right carotid artery ligation in neonates: classification of collateral flow with color Doppler imaging. Radiology. 1990 Apr;175(1):117-23.
24. Taylor GA, Short BL, Glass P, Ichord R, Cerebral hemodynamics in infants undergoing extracorporeal membrane oxygenation: further observations. *Radiology, July, 1988; 168, 163-167.*
25. Kolobow T, Zapol W, Pierce J. High survival and minimal blood damage in lambs exposed to long term (1 week) veno-venous pumping with a polyurethane chamber roller pump with and without a membrane oxygenator. Trans Am Soc Artif Intern Organs 1969; 15:172-177
26. Zwischenberger JB, Toomasian JM, Drake K, Andrews AF, Bartlett RH, Total respiratory support with single canula venovenous ECMO; double

lumen continuous flow vs. single lumen tidal flow ASAIO Trans 1985; 31:610-61
27. Sussmane JB, Totapally B, Hultquist K, Torbati D, Wolfsdorf J. Effects of arteriovenous extracorporeal therapy on hemodynamic stability, ventilation, and oxygenation in normal lambs. Crit Care Med 2001, 29(10): 1972-1978.
28. Burton G, Oxygen, the Janus effect; it's effects on human placental development and function, J. Anat 2009, July: 215(1): 27-35
29. Generation R, Eelhoed JJ. Steegers EA. van Osch-Gevers L. Verburg BO. Hofman A. Witteman JC. van der Heijden AJ. Helbing WA. Jaddoe VW., Cardiac Structures track during the first 2 years of life are associated with fetal growth and hemodynamics: American Heart Journal. 158(1):71-7, 2009 Jul.
30. Iserud T. Ebbing C. Kessler J. Rasmussen S Fetal cardiac output, distribution into the placenta and impact of placental compromise, Ultrasound in Obstetrics & Gynecology. 28(2):126-36, 2006 Aug.
31. Mielke G. Benda N., Cardiac output and central distribution of blood flow in the human fetus, Circulation. 103(12):1662-8, 2001 Mar 27.
32. Kakogawa J. Sumimoto K. Kawamura T. Minoura S. Kanayama N., Noninvasive monitoring of placental oxygenation by near-infrared spectroscopy, American Journal of Perinatology. 27(6):463-8, 2010 Jun.
33. Meschia G, Fetal Oxygenation and Maternal Ventilation Clinics in Chest Medicine, Vol. 32, Issue 1 March 2011
34. Virchow RLK, "Thrombose und Embolie. Gefässentzündung und septische Infektion." *Gesammelte Abhandlungen zur wissenschaftlichen Medicin*. Frankfurt am Main: Von Meidinger & Sohn. (1856). pp. 219-732. Translation in Matzdorff AC, Bell WR (1998). *Thrombosis and embolie (1846-1856)*. Canton, Massachusetts: Science History Publications. ISBN 0-88135-113-X.
35. Sussmane JB, Thrombotic Lesions of the Tricuspid Valve in the Newborn, Clin Peds, 1986; 25(4):225-27
36. Sussmane JB, Hematologic Considerations of Extracorporeal Life Support in Children, Int. J Pediatric Hematology/Oncology, 1994, Vol. 1:159-166
37. Fink SM, Bockman DE, Howell CG, et al, Bypass circuits as a source of thromboemboli during extracorporeal membrane oxygenation, J Pediatr, 1989: 621-624
38. Barrie WW, Wood EH, Crumlish P, Forbes CR, Prentice CRM, Low Dose Ancrod for the Prevention of Thrombotic Lesions after Surgery for Fractured Neck of Femur, 1974, BJM,4, 130-133

39. Shimada M, Matsumata T, Shirabe K, Kamakura T, Taketomi A, Sugimachi K, Effect of nafamostat mesilate on coagulation and fibrinolysis in hepatic resection, J. Am Coll Surg, May;178(5):498-502.
40. Shore, Lesserson et. al., TEG—Guided transfusion algorithm reduces transfusion in comlex cardiac surgery, Anesth Anal 1999,88:312-319
41. Carrmenzid V. et al, Thromboelastography, past present and future, Anesthesiology, 2000;92,1223-1226
42. Friday J, Kaplan A. Indications for therapeutic plasma exchange. Up-To-Date www.uptodateonline.com. Accessed January 13, 2005.
43. Madore F. Plasmapheresis: technical aspects and indications. *Crit Care Clin.* 2002; 8:375-392.
44. McMaster P., Shann F; The use of Extracorporeal Techniques to remove humoral factors in sepsis, Pediatr Crit Care med. 2003;30,4(1):2-7
45. Pisani E. Regulatory framework for plasmapheresis in the European Union: industry's viewpoint. *Hematology & Cell Therapy*, 1996, 38 Suppl 1:S35-
46. Clark WF, Rock GA, Buskard N, et.al. Therapeutic plasma exchange: An update from the Canadian Apheresis Group. *Ann Int Med.* 1999; 131:453-462.
47. Linenberger ML. Price TH. Use of cellular and plasma apheresis in the critically-ill patient: Part 1: technical and physiological considerations. *J Int Care Med.* 2005; 20:18-27.
48. Kellum JA, Venkataraman R. Blood purification in sepsis: an idea whose time has come. *Crit Care Med.* 2002; **30**:1387-1388.
49. Busund R, Koukline V, Utrobin U, et al. E Plasmapheresis in severe sepsis and septic shock: a prospective, randomised, controlled trial. *Int Care Med.* 2002; 28:1434-1439.
50. Custis, George Washington Parke, Recollections of Washington (1860); "The Death of George Washington, 1799"
51. Malchesky PS. Sueoka A. Matsubara S. et al. Membrane plasma separation. 1983. *Therapeutic Apheresis.* 2000; 4:47-53.
52. Yeh JH, Chen WH, Chiu HC. Complications of double-filtration plasmapheresis. *Transfusion.* 2004; 44:1621-1625.
53. Unger JK, Haltern C, Dohmen B, et al. Maximal flow rates and sieving coefficients in different plasmafilters: effects of increased membrane surfaces and effective length under standardized in vitro conditions. *J Clin Apheresis.* 2002; 17:190-198.
54. Gurland HJ, Lysaght MJ, Samtleben W, et al. A comparison of centrifugal and membrane-based apheresis formats. *Int J Artif Org.* 1984; 7:35-38.
55. Madore F. Plasmapheresis. Technical aspects and indications. *Crit Care Clinics.* 2002; 18:375-392.

56. DePalo T, Giordano M, Bellantuono, et al. Therapeutic apheresis in children, *Int J Artif Org.* 2000; 23:834-839.
57. Rock G, Buskard NA. Therapeutic plasmapheresis. *Curr Opin Hematol.* 1996; 3:504-510
58. Nenov VD, Marinov P, Sabeva J. Current applications of plasmapheresis in clinical toxicology. *Nephrol Dial Transp.* 2003; 18 Suppl 5:56-58.
59. Pond SM. Extracorporeal techniques in the treatment of poisoned patients. *Med J Aust.* 1991; 155:62-63.
60. Motohashi K, Yamane S. The effect of apheresis on adhesion molecules. Therapeutic Apheresis & Dialysis: Journal of the International Society for Apheresis, the Japanese Society for Apheresis, the Japanese Society for Dialysis Therapy. 2003; 7:425-430.
61. Gardlund B, Sjolin J, Nilsson A, et al. Plasma levels of cytokines in primary septic shock in humans: correlation with disease severity. *J Inf Dis.* 1995; **172**:296-301
62. Pisani BA, Mullen GM, Malinowska K, et.al, Plasmapheresis with intravenous immunoglobulin G is effective in patients with elevated panel reactive antibody prior to cardiac transplantation. *J Heart Lung Transplant.* 1999; 18:701-706.
63. Warren DS, Zachary AA, Sonnenday CJ,. et al. Successful renal transplantation across simultaneous ABO incompatible and positive crossmatch barriers. *Am J Transp.* 2004; 4:561-568.
64. Abraham KA, Brown C, Conlon PJ, et al. Plasmapheresis as rescue therapy in accelerated acute humoral rejection. *J Clin Apheresis.* 2003; 18:103-110.
65. Debray D, Furlan V, Baudoouin V, et. al, Therapy for acute rejection in pediatric organ transplant recipients. *Pediatr Drugs.* 2003; 5:81-93.
66. Stegmayr B. Plasmapheresis in severe sepsis or septic shock. *Blood Purif.* 1996; **14**:94-101.
67. McMaster P, Shann F. The use of extracorporeal techniques to remove humoral factors in sepsis. *Ped Crit Care Med.* 2003; 4:2-7.
68. Busund R, Koukline V, Utrobin U, et al. E Plasmapheresis in severe sepsis and septic shock: a prospective, randomised, controlled trial. *Int Care Med.* 2002; 28:1434-1439.
69. Felson DT, LaValley MP, Baldassare Ar, et al., The Prosorba column for the treatment of refractory rheumatoid arthritis: a randomized double-blind, sham-controlled trial. *Arthritis Rheum.* 1999; 42:2153-2159.
70. Aoki H, Kodama M, Tani T, et al. Treatment of sepsis by extracorporeal elimination of endotoxin using polymyxin B-immobilized fiber. *Am J Surg.* 1994; **167**:412-417.

71. Gorlin JB. Therapeutic plasma exchange and cytapheresis in pediatric patients. *Transfus Sci.* 1999; 21:21-39.
72. Urbaniak SJ. Therapeutic plasma and cellular apheresis. *Clinics in Haematology.* 1984; 13:217-251.
73. Grima KM. Therapeutic apheresis in hematological and oncological diseases. *J Clin Apheresis.* 2000; 15:28-52.
74. Kliman A, Carbone PP, Gaydos LA, et al. Effects of intensive plasmapheresis on normal blood donors. *Blood.* 1964; 23:647-656.
75. Pahl E, Crawford SE, Cohn RA, et al. Reversal of severe late left ventricular failure after pediatric heart transplantation and possible role of Plasmapheresis. *Am J Cardiol.* 2000; 85:735-739.
76. Berlot G, Tomasini A, Silvestri L, et al. Plasmapheresis in the critically-ill patient. Kidney International—Supplement. 1998; 66:S178-181.
77. Baldini GM, Silvestri MG, Quality Assurance in heampheresis: quality fresh frozen plasma, Int J Artif Organs, 1993;16, Suppl 5:226-228
78. Strauss RG. Apheresis donor safety—changes in humoral and cellular immunity. *J Clin Apheresis.* 1984; 2:68-80.
79. Sussmane J. Fifteen years of Plasmapheresis experience at Miami Children's Hospital. Int Peds 2009; 24(3):116-119.

Index

A

AaDO$_2$ (alveolar arterial difference of oxygen), 23
Abel, John Jacob, 16, 211
ACD-A, 184–85
albumin, 134
alteplase, 136
Amicar, 135
Anaximenes, 15
anticoagulation
 alternative therapies of, 137
Aprotinin, 132
argatroban, 136
AVDO$_2$ (arteriovenous oxygen difference), 30–31

B

BiVAD (biventricular assist device), 159
burbing, 101

C

cannulation
 blood gas management in, 102, 104
 and decannulation. See decannulation
 drug therapy of, 98
 fluid and electrolyte management in, 97–98
 heparin management in, 104
 membrane oxygenator monitoring in. See *under* membrane oxygenator
 nursing responsibilities in, 94
 O$_2$/CO$_2$ management in, 99–102
 patient management in, 95–97, 99
 and precannulation. See precannulation
 and trial-off periods. See trial-off stage
 VA bypass initiation in, 93–94
 VV-ECMO initiation in, 94
cardiopulmonary bypass, 29
CAVH-D (continuous arterial venous hemodiafiltration), 122–23
centrifuge, 176
clot formation, 128
CPS (cardiopulmonary support), 161–62
 in ECMO, 160
cryoprecipitate, 134
Ctesibius
 Pneumatica, 15
cytapheresis, 174

D

decannulation, 152–55, 156

DMAIC (define, measure, analyze, improve, and control), 49
DO$_2$ (oxygen delivery)
  factors, 38
  formula, 37

E

ECCO$_2$R (extracorporeal CO$_2$ removal), 43
ECLS (extracorporeal life support), 17
  perioperative cardiac support in, 158
  stinting in, 155–57
ECMO (extracorporeal membrane oxygenation)
  apheresis application in, 117–18
  arteriovenous, 19
  artificial placenta, 20–21
  blood product administration in, 130–37
  blood surface interactions in, 46
  competencies, 193–97
  complications of, 28
  definition of, 16–17
  flow factors in, 44–46
  indications and criteria in, 21
  outcomes of, 27
  patient care in, 108–13
  patient emergencies in, 160–69
  patient transportation in, 124–25
  physiology, 29–30
  specialist responsibilities in, 113–16
  special procedures in, 116
  VA (venoarterial), 17–18
  VV (veno-venous), 18–19
emergency decannulation, 162–63. See also decannulation
epsilon-aminocaproic acid. See Amicar

F

family-centered care, 176
FFP (fresh frozen plasma), 131
fibrin glue, 136, 165–66
Fick principle, 40
FiO$_2$ (fraction of inspired oxygen), 99

G

Galen, 174
Gibbon, John, 16, 212

H

hemofiltration, 113, 118, 120–21
hemoglobin oxygen disassociation curve, 32–37
Henry's law, 41
Hippocrates, 15, 211
HIT (heparin-induced thrombotic thrombocytopenia), 132, 136–37
Huang Di, 15, 174
  Neijing, 15

I

IABP (intra-aortic balloon pump), 158
in vivo occlusion setting protocol, 123–24

J

Jarvick, Robert, 16

K

Kolff, Willem Johan, 16, 211–12

L

leukopheresis, 174

LMWH (low molecular weight heparin), 137
Lomoparin, 137
Lower, Richard
  Tractatus de Corde, 15
LVAD (left ventricular assist device), 159

M

membrane oxygenator
  definition of, 17
  monitoring, 105–8
  oxygen transfer formula of, 107
membrane ventilating gas flow. See sweep flow
MVO_2 (mixed venous saturation), 40–43

N

Neijing (Huang Di), 15, 211

O

oxygen
  consumption. See VO_2 (oxygen consumption)
  content, 30–31
  delivery. See DO_2 (oxygen delivery)
  independent metabolism, 41

P

packed red blood cells. See PRBCs (packed red blood cells)
patient-centered care, 51
plasmapheresis, 16, 174
  competencies, 189–90
  complications of, 214
  ECMO circuit considerations in, 177
  fluid balance formula of, 183
  humoral considerations in, 178–79
  nursing care in, 187–88
  physiologic considerations in, 180–83
  principles of, 175–77
  responsibilities of, 177
plasmin, 135
platelets, 131–33
Pneumatica (Ctesibius), 15
pneumatic chemistry, 15
Poiseuille's law, 105
PRBCs (packed red blood cells), 130
precannulation
  admission orders in, 87–91
  circuit priming process of, 60–84
  evaluation, 54–55
  medical preparations of, 85–87
  process, 55–59
  safety checklist of, 60
process (definition), 49

Q

quality
  functional, 50
  perceived, 50
  technical, 48, 50

R

rated flow, 101
rATIII (recombinant antithrombin III), 136
r-tPA (recombinant tissue-type plasminogen activator). See alteplase
RVAD (right ventricular assist device), 159

S

SERVQUAL, 51
Six Sigma, 49
sweep flow, 43, 99–101

T

TEG (thromboelastogram), 137
thesbian flow, 46
TPE (therapeutic plasma exchange). See plasmapheresis
TQM (total quality management), 49
Tractatus de Corde (Lower), 15
trial-off stage, 150, 152

V

VAD (ventricular assist device), 158–59
ventilator, 17
Virchow, 126, 164
VO_2 (oxygen consumption), 40–42

W

weaning and idling
   open-bridge ECMO, 148–50
   VV-ECMO, 150–51

Y

Yellow Emperor's Classic of Medicine. See *Neijing* (Huang Di)

www.ingramcontent.com/pod-product-compliance
Lightning Source LLC
Chambersburg PA
CBHW030925180526
45163CB00002B/468